Guide to Your Natural Well-being

Conscious Choices for a Balanced Life, Transform Your Life in Small Steps

Volume 1

By
Linda Welsh
and
Antonio Mens

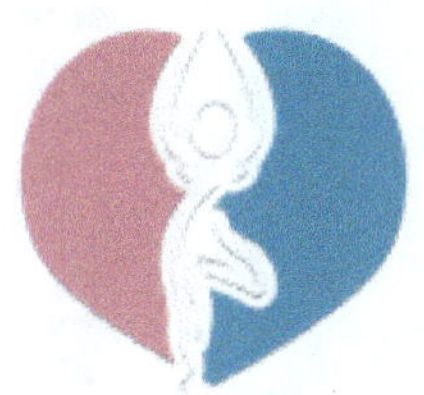

Book Series
"Sana Vitae"

First edition

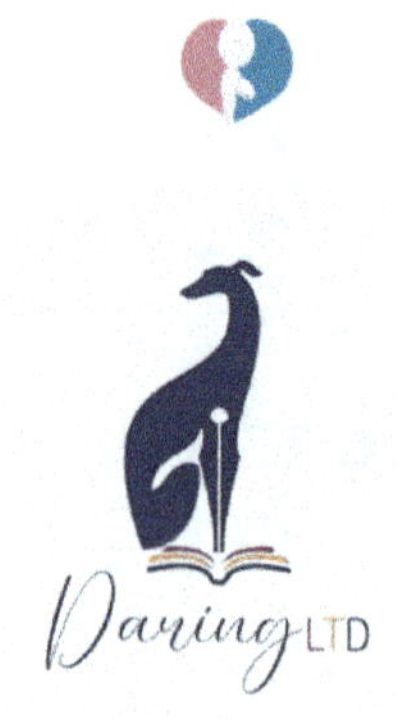

Content

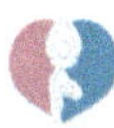

Disclamer

"No guide or advice contained in these pages should ever be interpreted as an alternative to official medical treatments. Modern medicine, with its vast repertoire of knowledge, is essential for addressing specific medical conditions, diagnosing diseases, and providing targeted treatments. Under no circumstances should the information contained herein be interpreted as a substitute for professional medical consultation."

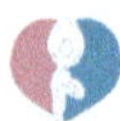

Authors' Biography

Linda Welch, born and raised in the picturesque countryside of Italy, has always had a deep connection with nature and a passionate spirit for promoting well-being. With a degree in Natural Sciences, Linda has dedicated her life to exploring and understanding the healing power of nature. Her interest in mindful eating and healthy lifestyles led her to collaborate with her husband, Antonio Mens, in creating a comprehensive guide to natural well-being.

Antonio Mens, coming from a family of medical professionals, has always had a passion for science and research. With a degree in Medicine, Antonio developed a profound understanding of the dynamics of the human body and the importance of a healthy lifestyle. His experience in the medical field, combined with his vision of a balanced life, harmoniously merged with his wife Linda Welch's perspective, creating a unique collaboration aimed at guiding people towards conscious choices for a balanced life.

"Sana Vitae" is a series dedicated to exploring and sharing secrets and practices for a healthy and harmonious lifestyle. Through approaches based on science, intuition, and ancient wisdom, Linda Welch and Antonio Mens offer a comprehensive journey to discover natural well-being. Each book in the series is designed to inspire, educate, and motivate readers to make conscious choices for a balanced life.

The books of "Sana Vitae" are the answer to the growing desire for an authentic and reliable guide in the field of well-being, providing practical tools and wisdom that transform theory into action for lasting well-being.

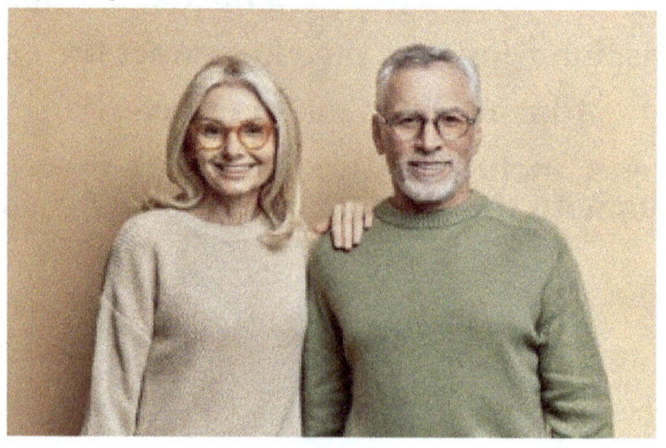

 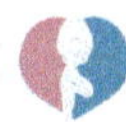

Premise

There is a saying that goes: "Every journey begins with a single step," and today you have taken that step. I am thrilled to share with you tips, secrets, and a bit of wisdom that will make your journey toward well-being a special and fulfilling experience. Are you ready to embark on a journey towards natural well-being and optimal health?

Welcome to the "Guide to Natural Well-being," a reliable companion that explores conscious choices to shape a balanced life. This book is an invitation to explore alternative and complementary approaches to improve your well-being. It is not a complicated manual or a list of rigid rules but an invitation to explore how small changes can make a big difference in your daily life. Know that this is just the beginning of your well-being adventure!

We live in an era where access to information is unprecedented, allowing us to explore a vast array of options to improve our health and well-being. The "Guide to Natural Well-being" aims to be a compass on this journey, offering practical advice, ancient wisdom, and modern insights to help you shape a healthier and more balanced lifestyle.

The heart of this book is the promotion of conscious choices. From how we nourish ourselves to stress management, from connecting with nature to caring for our body and mind, we will explore a wide range of topics aimed at providing practical tools for personal improvement. However, it is imperative to emphasize that the information presented here is for guidance and should not replace the advice of qualified medical professionals.

The "Guide to Natural Well-being" is for those interested in exploring integrative approaches to improving their health. It is for those open to discovering the wonders of herbal medicine, healthy eating, balanced physical activity, and stress management practices. However, it is important to note that this book is not intended for those seeking definitive answers or miracle cures without a professional medical approach.

Each individual is unique, and the path to well-being is inherently personal. What works for one person may not be the perfect solution for another. The "Guide to Natural Well-being" is designed to provide a general framework of healthy

 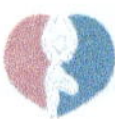

practices, but adaptation and personalization are essential. It is always advisable to consult a medical professional before making significant lifestyle changes or embarking on new health regimens.

This is the first volume of an extraordinary series, so prepare for further volumes that will explore intriguing topics and practical tips to improve various aspects of your life. Each volume will be a new chapter in our journey together towards deeper and lasting well-being.

Ultimately, this book is conceived as a companion for exploration in the world of natural well-being. It is an invitation to be mindful of the daily choices that shape our health, with the important caveat that official medicine is irreplaceable when it comes to specific treatments. Whether you are starting your journey towards a healthier life or seeking new perspectives to improve your well-being, know that your health is a treasure and that taking care of yourself is an act of love and respect towards your life.

Immagine freepik.com

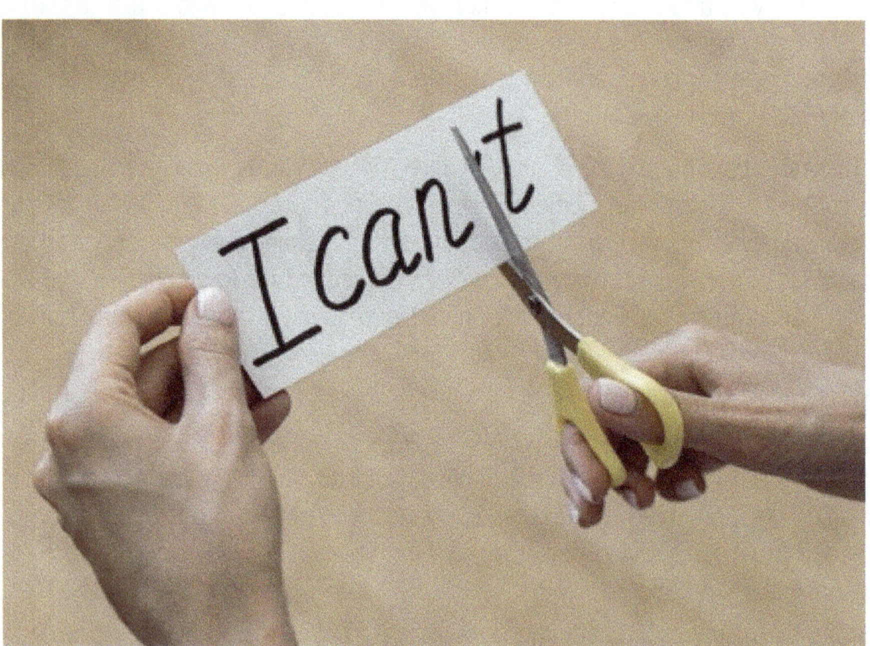

 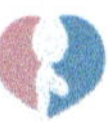

Chapter 1: The Benefit of Seven Evening Habits

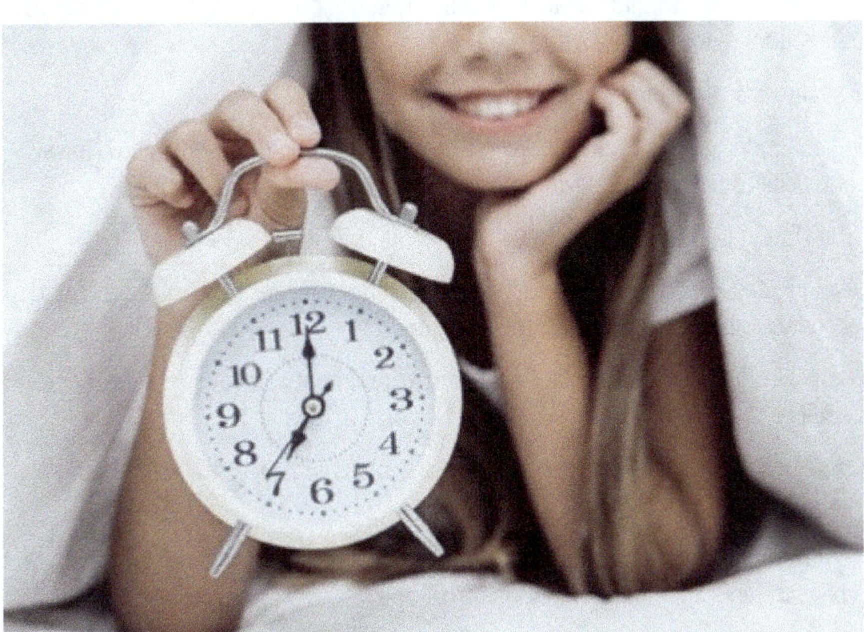

I firmly believe that, especially during youth, we tend to underestimate the incredible power of habits. They are not just routines that shape our day, but they influence our physical appearance, our health, and even our identity and way of being.

In the evening, when the sun sets, and the day draws to a close, it becomes essential to slow down, allowing the body and mind to relax.

The evening habits you maintain can have a significant impact on the quality of your sleep and your energy upon waking. I want to guide you through this journey, helping you create habits that promote well-being.

Let's now understand the power of seven evening habits that have a potent impact on your nighttime routines, the quality of your sleep, and your overall well-being.

Often, the mistake is made of stimulating the mind until feeling exhausted, extending evenings longer than necessary. If the usual bedtime is around 9:30 or 10:00 PM, it's common to find oneself procrastinating until late at night, compromising sleep.

 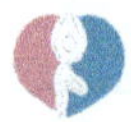

Examine your current evening habits to understand how they affect your nightly sleep and realize the importance of making conscious changes to improve your routine and ensure restful sleep.

First Habit: Preparing for Relaxation Before Bed

One common habit is to start relaxing only when it's time to go to bed. However, it is crucial to begin the relaxation process a few hours before bedtime.

- Start Early: Educate your body to relax around 7:30-8:00 PM.

- Avoid Excessive Stimulation: Reduce stimulating activities and opt for a light dinner to facilitate a smooth transition to sleep.

- Natural Light: Avoid artificial lights and experiment with the relaxing effect of candlelight.

Besides changing your evening approach, it is essential to create a relaxing routine before bed.

- Serene Activities: Read a book, listen to relaxing music, or practice meditation to prepare your mind and emotions for sleep.

- Consistency and Commitment: Changing your habits takes time, but once integrated, they will improve your sleep and overall well-being.

I urge you to reflect on these dynamics and adopt healthier habits for your evening routine. Conscious management of your nighttime habits will lead to more restful sleep and a more energetic wake-up. Be patient, consistent, and embrace the change. The benefits will be enormous, even influencing your character and how you approach life.

Second Habit: Clearing the Mind Before Bed

One habit that can negatively affect your sleep is carrying the day's worries with you. Often, the mind remains active, incessantly ruminating on what you need to face the next day. To address this situation, it is essential to learn to manage your worries and clear your mind before going to bed.

- Keep a Notebook or Planner: Create a safe space to jot down the next day's activities.

- Save Time in the Morning: Review and update your task list before bed to offload recurring thoughts.

- Clarity and Organization: Write down your activities in detail so they are easy to consult the next day.

- Relaxation Sessions: Spend a few minutes before bed to mentally and emotionally relax.

- Meditation or Deep Breathing: Practice short sessions to release the tensions accumulated during the day.

- Consistency in Notebook Use: Maintain the practice of using the notebook consistently to gain maximum benefits.

- Necessary Updates: Update the task list as needed, ensuring a clear and calm mind before bed.

The goal of this habit is to teach you to free your mind from unnecessary thoughts and worries, creating a serene and calm mental space before bed. Cultivating the habit of writing down your activities and dedicating time to relaxation can make a big difference in the quality of your sleep and overall well-being.

Remember, even though there may be initial resistance, consistency will bring positive changes. Over time, you will notice a reduction in anxiety and an improvement in the quality of your sleep. Keep practicing these habits, experiment with what works best for you, and enjoy the benefits of a clear mind and more restful sleep.

Third Habit: Cultivating Evening Optimism

Going to bed with a pessimistic mindset can negatively affect your sleep and mood. In this third habit, we will explore how you can change your perspective before going to bed by embracing a more optimistic attitude.

- Positive Attitude: Consider the importance of adopting an optimistic attitude before going to sleep.

- Reflect on Positive Aspects: Take a moment to reflect on the positive events of the day.

- List of Positive Things: Make a brief mental list of the positive experiences of the day.

 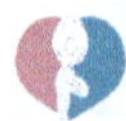

- Journal Writing: Write in a journal about the things you are grateful for each evening.

- Focus on Positive Moments: Concentrate on joys, successes, and kind gestures to shift attention from negative thoughts.

- Positive Evening Routine: Dedicate time to meditation, inspirational reading, or listening to relaxing music.

- Let Go of Pessimism: Release negative thoughts and worries, fostering a serene and optimistic state of mind.

- Regular Exercises: Practice regularly listing positive things before bed.

- Gradual Integration: Experiment with different activities that promote positive thoughts to find what works best for you.

Changing this habit requires time and consistency. However, as the weeks go by, you will notice an improvement in your sleep and overall well-being. Cultivating an optimistic mindset can lead to greater mental tranquility, contributing to more restorative sleep.

Remember to be patient with yourself during this process of change. Experiment and observe how optimism can positively influence your sleep quality. Over time, you will enjoy the benefits of a positive mindset and more restful sleep.

Fourth Habit: An Evening Without Intense Emotions

Going to bed after watching a movie, a game, or a competition can compromise the quality of your sleep. In this fourth habit, we will explore how to manage evening activities that evoke intense emotions and how to create an evening more conducive to relaxation.

Reflection on Managing Evening Emotions

- Effect of Intense Emotions: Discover how intense emotions can affect your breathing and mood before bed.

- Preparing the Mind for Sleep: Choose relaxing activities that promote a smooth transition to sleep.

Modifying the Evening Routine

 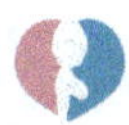

- Avoid Stimulating Activities: Opt for less intense activities like reading or meditation.

- Dedicated Relaxation Time: Spend at least an hour before bed engaging in relaxing activities.

- Reduce Electronic Device Use: Avoid stimulating devices at least an hour before bed.

Considerations for the Nighttime Environment

- Bedroom Temperature: Ensure your bedroom is at a comfortable temperature.

- Eliminate Blue Light: Avoid intense artificial lights before bed to not interfere with melatonin production.

Evening Relaxation Techniques

- Deep Breathing: Practice slow, deep breathing exercises to calm the mind.

- Yoga or Meditation: Integrate practices that induce a state of relaxation.

Time and Consistency for Adapting to Changes

- Gradual Progress: Understand that changing habits takes time and consistency.

- Observe Changes: Pay attention to how these modifications affect your sleep quality.

- Adapt the Routine: Experiment with different activities to find what works best for you.

Insight on Breathing and Sleep

- Nighttime Breathing Exercises: Practice specific exercises before bed to promote deep, regular breathing.

Changing this habit can lead to a smoother transition to sleep and more restorative rest. With time and consistent practice, you can enjoy the benefits of an evening free from intense emotions, setting the stage for more peaceful and satisfying sleep.

Fifth Habit: Nasal Breathing for Restorative Sleep

The fifth habit focuses on breathing, an often overlooked but crucial element for quality sleep. Mouth breathing can compromise your physical well-being and sleep

 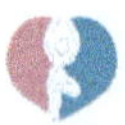

quality. In this section, we will explore how to adopt nasal breathing for more restorative rest.

The Importance of Nasal Breathing

- Optimal Nature of Nasal Breathing: Understand why nasal breathing is fundamental for physical well-being and sleep.

- Risks of Mouth Breathing: Learn how mouth breathing can cause sleep apnea and airway obstructions.

Experimenting with Nasal Breathing Practices

- Nasal Breathing Exercises: Practice specific exercises, such as inhaling deeply through the nose and exhaling slowly through the mouth.

- Saline Solutions or Nasal Sprays: Use saline solutions to reduce swelling and promote clear airways.

Patience and Consistency for Change

- Gradual Adaptation: Understand that change takes time, especially if you have established breathing habits.

- Daily Persistence: Continue to motivate yourself to breathe through the nose daily, even if it initially seems difficult.

Insight on Nighttime Breathing

- Progress and Adaptation: Over time, your physiology will gradually adapt, improving nasal breathing and, consequently, sleep quality.

- Consult a Professional: If persistent difficulties arise, consider consulting a doctor or sleep specialist.

Integrate Changes into the Evening Routine

- Evening Breathing: Dedicate a moment in the evening to practice breathing exercises before bed.

- Create a Favorable Environment: Ensure your bedroom is cool and comfortable to facilitate nasal breathing.

Final Reflection on Nasal Breathing

 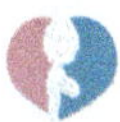

Adopting nasal breathing as a nighttime habit can bring numerous benefits to your overall health and sleep quality. With consistency and commitment, you can enjoy the advantages of proper nasal breathing, contributing to more restful and restorative sleep.

Sixth Habit: The Influence of Hormones in the Falling Asleep Process

In this sixth habit, we explore the importance of hormones in regulating sleep and how you can incorporate evening practices to promote a more natural and restorative falling asleep process.

The Magic of Hormones for Your Evening Relaxation

Hormones play a magical role in promoting evening relaxation and well-being, creating an elegant chemical symphony that prepares your body for the night. Let's discover together the key role these chemical messengers play in contributing to your evening serenity.

Let's delve into how hormones play a crucial role in regulating sleep and overall body balance:

Sleep is much more than a simple rest period; it's an intricate ballet orchestrated by the hormones in your body. These chemical messengers play a crucial role in regulating sleep and maintaining overall body balance. Let's explore the role of some of these key players and how they can influence your sleep quality.

Melatonin is often called the "sleep hormone." This chemical, produced by the pineal gland in the brain, regulates the circadian rhythm. It increases as light decreases, preparing your body for sleep. Reducing exposure to blue light from screens before bed can improve melatonin production, promoting deeper sleep.

Cortisol, also known as the stress hormone, plays a crucial role in maintaining energy and alertness during the day. However, high cortisol levels at night can disturb sleep. Practicing stress management, such as meditation or deep breathing, can help keep cortisol under control.

Serotonin is involved in regulating mood and sleep. It transforms into melatonin in your brain, setting the stage for sleep. Foods rich in tryptophan, a precursor to serotonin, like turkey and bananas, can promote the production of this chemical.

Ghrelin and Leptin: These two hormones are not directly linked to sleep but their balance affects appetite and body weight, which in turn can impact sleep.

 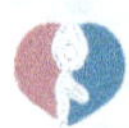

Maintaining a healthy body weight through a balanced diet and exercise can help regulate ghrelin and leptin.

Growth Hormone is primarily released during the deepest stages of sleep. This hormone supports growth, cell repair, and overall health. Ensure you get enough sleep to maximize the benefits of this valuable hormone.

In adults, reproductive hormones like estrogens and progesterone can influence sleep quality, especially in women during the menstrual cycle and menopause. Medical advice and self-care practices can help manage hormonal fluctuations to improve sleep.

Oxytocin, often called the love or hug hormone, is involved in regulating emotions and social bonding. Hugs, affectionate gestures, and positive physical contact can increase oxytocin levels, contributing to your relaxed emotional state and creating a pleasant evening atmosphere.

Dopamine, involved in motivation and pleasure, can enhance your evening entertainment. Activities that bring joy and satisfaction, such as listening to favorite music or engaging in a beloved hobby, can stimulate dopamine, improving your overall well-being.

Endorphins, often called the "happiness hormones," are released during physical exercise and pleasurable situations. Even a simple smile or laughter can increase endorphins, contributing to your happy and relaxed evening.

Understanding how hormones contribute to your evening relaxation gives you the opportunity to direct your own well-being symphony. With mindful practices such as pre-sleep relaxation, stress management, and emotional nourishment, you can harmonize hormones to create an evening experience that promotes sleep and overall well-being. May your night be a magical representation of tranquility and rest.

Restorative sleep is the result of harmony between various hormones in your body. Maintaining a healthy hormonal balance requires a combination of lifestyle practices such as a balanced diet, regular exercise, and stress management strategies. Listening to your body's signals and adopting habits that promote hormonal balance can lead to more restful nights and improved overall well-being.

Wrap Yourself in Warmth: A Warm Ritual for Your Evening

 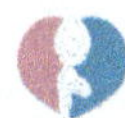

Incorporating warm elements into your evening routine is a cozy way to prepare your body and mind for a night of restorative rest. Let's explore together how warmth can become a touching ritual in your evening.

Integrating a cup of warm tea into your evening is not just a gesture but an act of self-love. Herbs like chamomile, lavender, or peppermint can have relaxing effects, helping to calm the nerves and prepare you for sleep. The enveloping warmth of a hot drink becomes a meditative ritual, allowing you to disconnect from the tensions of the day.

Experiencing a warm shower or bath is like immersing yourself in a sanctuary of warmth and relaxation. Warm water helps to dissolve accumulated muscle tension, releasing physical and mental fatigue. You can enhance this experience by adding essential oils like lavender or peppermint oil to boost the relaxing effects and create an enveloping atmosphere.

Warm water not only soothes the body but also has a therapeutic power. You can turn this moment into a self-care ritual, allowing the water to wash away stress and prepare you for a deep rest. Add a few drops of lavender essential oil or scented bath salts to your bath to amplify the calming effect.

Hydration is an essential part of your evening ritual. Sipping a cup of warm water can be a mindfulness practice, a moment when you pay attention to your body. You can enrich the water with citrus slices or a splash of ginger for a refreshing and nourishing touch.

In addition to physical warmth, warm lighting plays a crucial role in your evening. Use softer, warmer lights in the hours leading up to sleep to signal your body that it's time to relax. The cozy atmosphere will help calm your mind, preparing it for a peaceful sleep.

Incorporating warm elements into your evening routine is like wrapping your body and soul in a nightly embrace. This ritual not only improves sleep quality but also creates a space for your inner peace. Indulge in these moments of warmth to find balance and live your night serenely.

Activate Your Parasympathetic System for Relaxation

Stimulating the parasympathetic system through warmth is key to promoting a sense of deep relaxation. Let's discover together how this simple gesture can become a therapeutic embrace for your mind and body.

 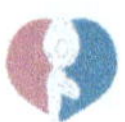

The parasympathetic system is the counterpart of the sympathetic nervous system, often activated during moments of stress and intense activity. Stimulating the parasympathetic system is like pressing the reset button for your body, inducing a state of relaxation and calm.

Warmth has a direct effect on the nervous system's response, especially when targeted at key areas of the body. Warm baths, warm showers, or even warm compresses can activate the parasympathetic system, inducing a relaxation response.

Stimulating the Parasympathetic System with Heat

Stimulating the parasympathetic system through heat is key to promoting a sense of deep relaxation. Let's discover together how this simple gesture can become a therapeutic embrace for your mind and body.

The parasympathetic system is the counterpart of the sympathetic nervous system, often activated during moments of stress and intense activities. Stimulating the parasympathetic system is like pressing the reset button for your body, inducing a state of relaxation and calm.

Heat has a direct effect on the nervous system's response, especially when targeted to key areas of the body. Hot baths, hot showers, or even hot compresses can activate the parasympathetic system, inducing a relaxation response that spreads throughout the body.

When you immerse your body in a hot shower or soak in a hot bath, you are creating a ritual of calm and tranquility. This is not only a moment to cleanse the physical body but also to melt away mental tensions and worries. The heat becomes the vehicle that takes you into a state of serenity.

We live in a world where frenzy is often the norm. Stimulating the parasympathetic system through heat is a revolutionary act of slowing down. It is like telling your body to take the time to regenerate, to honor the need for calm in a world that often seems accelerated.

Combine the experience of heat with a practice of mindful breathing. Breathe deeply, allowing the heat to penetrate deeply into your body. Exhale slowly, releasing accumulated tensions. The combination of heat and mindful breathing is a powerful blend for activating the parasympathetic system.

 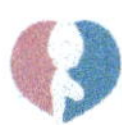

Including heat in your routine is more than just a physical act; it is a warm embrace for your mental and physical health. Allow yourself this daily gesture of warmth, and feel how your parasympathetic system responds with gratitude, bringing you into a state of deep relaxation.

Considerations on Bedroom Temperature:

Often overlooked, the temperature of your bedroom plays a fundamental role in the quality of your sleep. Let's explore together why you should pay attention to this often overlooked detail.

The ambient temperature of your bedroom can significantly influence your ability to fall asleep and stay asleep. A cool temperature, ideally around 18-20 degrees Celsius, creates a comfortable environment and promotes relaxation.

While it may seem tempting, an overly warm environment can compromise your sleep quality. High temperatures can lead to sweating and discomfort, disturbing the natural sleep cycle and reducing the depth of rest.

Thermal comfort is subjective, but generally, a cool temperature promotes a sense of coziness and comfort. A well-ventilated room with the right temperature creates the ideal conditions for restorative sleep.

- Adequate Ventilation: Ensure that your bedroom is well-ventilated to guarantee a flow of fresh air.

- Use of Light Blankets: Prefer light blankets that allow for more precise temperature regulation.

- Breathable Materials: Use sheets and blankets made of breathable materials to avoid overheating.

Every individual is unique, and personal temperature preferences can vary. Listen to your body and adjust your bedroom temperature according to your personal needs to ensure a peaceful and restorative night of sleep.

Your bedroom is the sanctuary of sleep, and temperature plays a crucial role in promoting quality rest. With a few practical adjustments, you can create a cozy environment that cradles your body during the night and prepares you for a rejuvenated day.

In-depth Look at Hormonal Regulation

 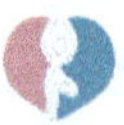

Hormonal regulation is a fundamental part of maintaining balance in your body. In this in-depth look, we will explore how heat can become an ally in stimulating hormones that promote relaxation and prepare the ground for restorative sleep.

Experimenting with heat consciously can positively influence hormonal regulation. Some practices to consider include:

A hot shower or relaxing bath before bed can raise body temperature and promote melatonin production, preparing the body for quality sleep.

Moderate exposure to sunlight during the day can stimulate the production of vitamin D, an important hormonal regulator associated with well-being and the immune system.

Heat exposure in these structures can trigger a relaxing response, stimulating the production of wellness-related hormones.

Exploring variations in temperature between hot and cold during the day can modulate your hormonal response, creating a beneficial adaptation effect. Some practices include:

Alternating between hot and cold water during the shower can improve blood circulation, stimulate the immune system, and promote vitality.

Every individual is unique, and the body's response to heat can vary. Listening carefully to your body is essential. While these practices can be beneficial for many, it is important to personalize them according to your individual needs and sensations.

Harnessing heat to regulate hormones is a practical and natural approach to improving your overall well-being. By consciously integrating heat into your daily routine, you can create a space of relaxation and prepare the ground for restorative sleep. Listen to your body and embrace the beneficial power of heat in your daily life.

Integrating warm elements into your evening routine can help stimulate relaxation and facilitate the process of falling asleep. With time and consistency, you will be able to appreciate the benefits of an evening routine that naturally supports the work of hormones for more restful sleep.

 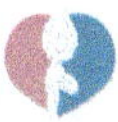

Seventh Habit: Considering the Impact of Daily Activities on Sleep

The seventh habit focuses on how daily activities influence your nighttime sleep. Establishing a consistent routine during the day can play a crucial role in promoting restorative sleep. Let's explore how to structure the day to improve the quality of your nighttime rest.

- Importance of Routine: Understand how a consistent routine helps regulate your biological clock.

- Impact on Sleep Quality: Recognize how consistency in daily habits can positively influence nighttime sleep.

- Stability in Wake-Up and Bedtime: Adopt the habit of waking up and going to bed at the same time every day.

- Creating a Morning Ritual: Implement a series of consistent activities every morning to start the day positively.

- Incorporating Physical Exercise: Integrate physical activity into your day, but avoid intense efforts just before bedtime. Practicing outdoor activities in different weather conditions, when possible, can expose the body to a range of temperatures, contributing to its adaptability.

- Optimal Workout Times: Choose specific times during the day to exercise, such as in the morning or early afternoon.

- Regularity in Meals: Maintain regular times for main meals to stabilize your metabolism.

- Avoiding Heavy Meals Before Sleep: Reduce food intake in the hours close to nighttime rest to facilitate digestion.

- Reflect on How Daily Activities Impact Your Sleep: Organize the evening with quiet activities to prepare the body and mind for rest.

- Long-Term Benefits: Recognize how a consistent routine can influence your mental and physical health.

- Anxiety and Panic Symptoms: Understand how stability in daily habits can help reduce anxiety and panic attacks.

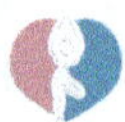

- Observe and Adapt: Experiment with a consistent daily routine and observe how it affects sleep quality.

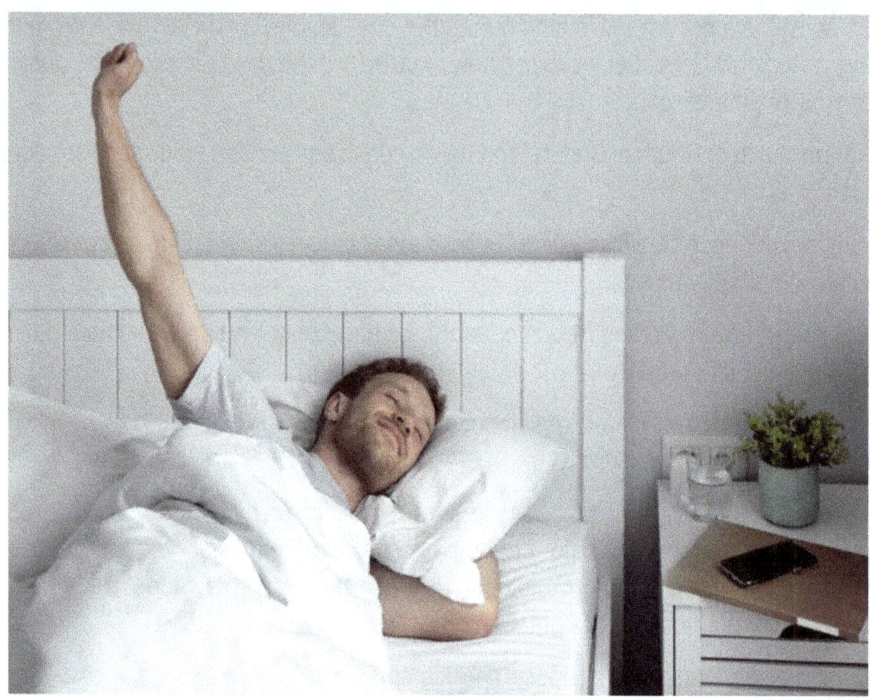

- Persistence in Implementing Changes: Recognize that consistency is key to achieving long-term benefits.

Considering the impact of daily activities on sleep is essential to ensure a consistent routine that supports your overall well-being. Experiment with structuring the day and adjust habits according to your needs, contributing to more restful and regenerative sleep.

 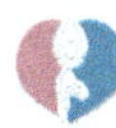

Chapter 2: Five Breathing Exercises to Nourish Your Body and Mind

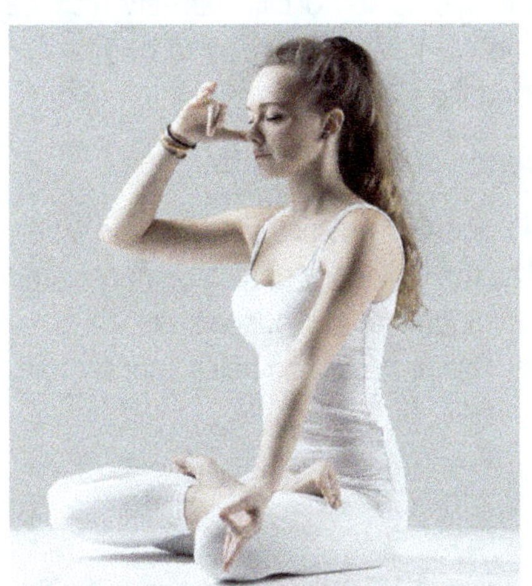

 Here we are at the second chapter of our journey towards well-being. I am so happy that you are continuing this path of exploration and self-discovery. Now, we will talk about something fundamental: the connection between mind and body. I have gained a lot of experience over the years, and I want to share my knowledge with you on how your thoughts can directly impact your physical health.

The Dance Between Mind and Body

Scientific research clearly supports the importance of breathing for our mental and physical health. Regularly integrating breathing exercises into your daily routine is not just an act of self-care but a practice supported by science that can positively transform your life.

I invite you to consider these breathing exercises as powerful tools for your overall well-being. Science confirms that dedicating even just a few minutes a day to these practices can have lasting impacts on your mental and physical health. Breathe deeply and start this small yet powerful transformation today. Your health will thank you.

Numerous scientific studies have confirmed the deep connection between mind and body, emphasizing how thoughts and emotions directly influence our physiology. A study published in the Journal of Clinical Psychology highlighted that negative thoughts can contribute to stress conditions, which in turn can manifest with physical symptoms such as muscle tension and gastrointestinal disturbances.

Perhaps you have noticed, as I have, that when thoughts are dark and pessimistic, the body responds with inflammation, stiffness, and contraction. Conversely, a stressed body can trigger anxiety, depression, and even panic attacks. It is an intricate dance between the head and the heart, and understanding this connection is the first step towards improving your life.

The Five Magical Breathing Exercises

 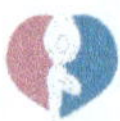

Let's explore together five breathing exercises that you can integrate into your morning routine. They are like little daily magic spells to calm anxiety, reduce stress, and bring you into the present moment. I have been inspired by years of study and working with people like you, facing life's challenges.

4-2 / 4-2 Breathing Exercise: The Science of Deep Breathing

The 4-2 / 4-2 breathing exercise is a deep breathing practice, a technique widely supported by research. A study conducted by the University of Pisa demonstrated that deep breathing can activate the parasympathetic nervous system, thus reducing stress and promoting a state of calm. This practice also helps improve lung function by increasing lung capacity.

Here's how to proceed:

- Inhale slowly for 4 seconds.

- Hold your breath for 2 seconds.

- Exhale gently for 4 seconds.

- Remain without air for 2 seconds.

- Repeat. This practice calms the mind and promotes deep breathing.

1. Lip Breathing: An Ancient Relaxation Technique

The lip breathing exercise is a relaxation technique rooted in meditation practices. Studies conducted at Harvard University have shown that relaxation through breathing can reduce levels of cortisol, the stress hormone, in the body. This suggests that practices like lip breathing can be effective in managing stress.

Here's how to proceed:

- Inhale through your nose, filling your lungs.

- Exhale slowly through slightly pursed lips, imagining blowing out a candle.

- Develop deep and mindful breathing.

2. Bee Breath: Connection Between Sound and Tranquility

The bee breath exercise, engaging with its buzzing sound, finds support in the psychology of sound. A study from Stanford University found that exposure to relaxing sounds can activate the parasympathetic nervous system, leading to a

 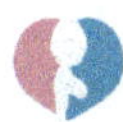

reduction in stress. The controlled emission of sound during the bee breath exercise can have calming benefits for the mind.

Here's how to proceed:

- Gently place your fingers on your ears.

- Inhale, then exhale while making a humming sound like a bee (mmmmmmmmmmmm).

- Focus on the sound to bring tranquility and peace.

3. Alternate Nostril Breathing: Balance Through Breathing

The alternate nostril breathing exercise is an ancient yoga practice, but its validity is supported by modern science. A study published in the Journal of Ayurveda and Integrative Medicine indicated that this technique can balance brain activities and reduce anxiety. Breathing through one nostril can influence specific regions of the brain, leading to greater emotional balance.

Here's how to proceed:

- Gently cover one nostril with your finger and inhale.

- Switch sides and exhale through the other nostril.

- This exercise promotes relaxation and body awareness.

4. Energizing Breath: Stimulate Energy Through Breathing

The energizing breath exercise finds support in research on vigorous breathing. A study from the University of Adelaide demonstrated that vigorous breathing can increase energy levels and improve vitality. This powerful exercise can be particularly beneficial in countering feelings of fatigue and apathy.

Here's how to proceed:

- Inhale through your nose, then forcefully exhale repeatedly.

- You can press your hands on your knees for added strength.

- This exercise stimulates energy and enhances vitality.

I encourage you to dedicate a few minutes each morning to these breathing exercises. It will be your moment of intimacy with yourself, an opportunity to calm the mind and nourish the body. Day by day, you will notice the difference. You will feel calmer, less stressed, and more aware.

When we learn to control our breath, we influence our thoughts, our mind, and reduce anxiety and stress. Remember, even a few minutes a day dedicated to yourself can make a big difference. Continue this practice and observe how your life transforms for the better.

I am excited to continue this journey together. Breathe deeply and start this small yet powerful transformation today.

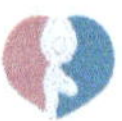

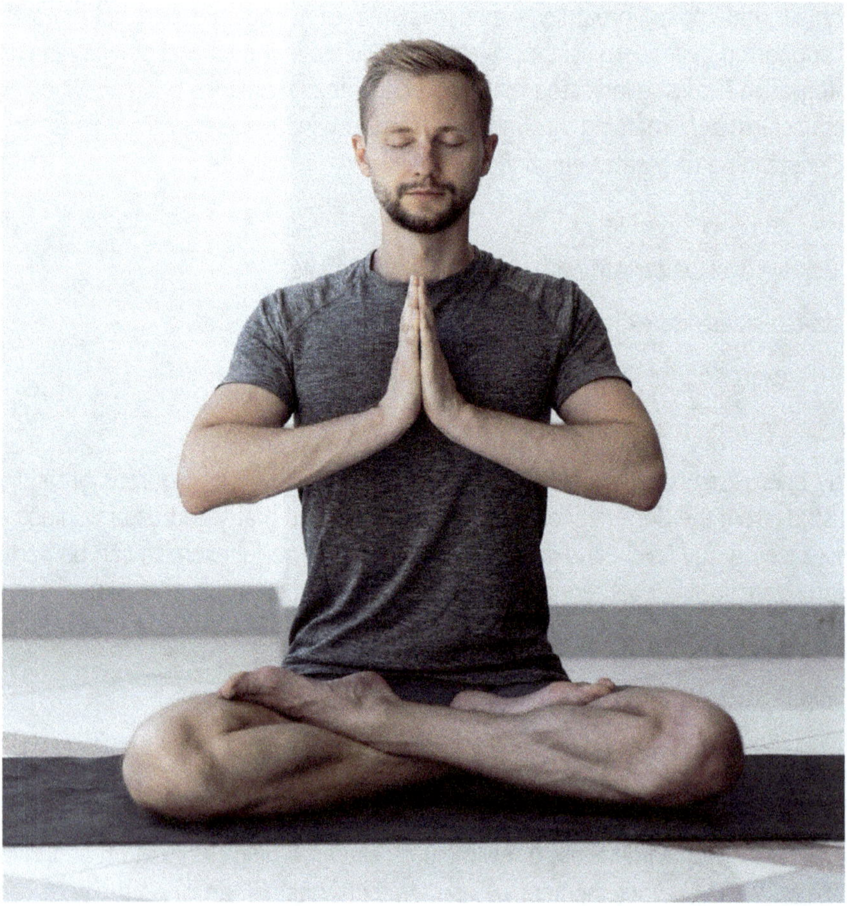

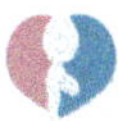

Chapter 3: Discover the Benefits of Taking a Cold Shower Every Day

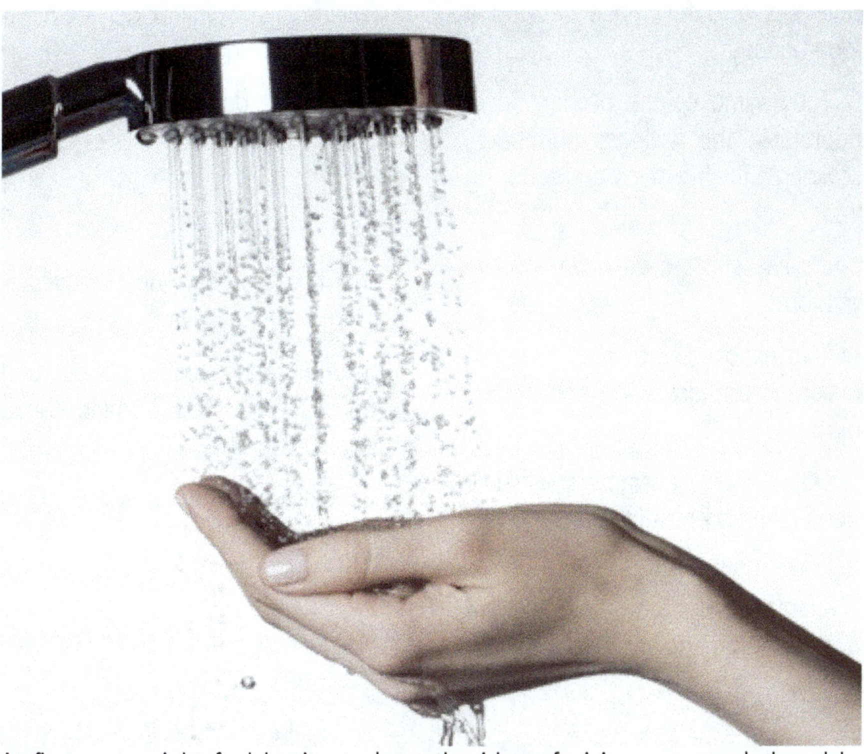

At first, you might feel hesitant about the idea of giving up your beloved hot shower, but let me explain the reasons why this practice can transform your overall well-being.

The wonderful benefits of taking a daily cold shower might seem a bit intimidating at first, but trust me, the advantages you'll gain will be absolutely worth it. Get ready to explore a new world of energy, vitality, and well-being!

1. Increase in Energy and Vitality:

- Exposure to cold during the shower is like a wake-up call for your body.

- It stimulates blood circulation and activates the sympathetic nervous system.

- The result? A tangible increase in energy and vitality that will accompany you throughout the day.

2. Mood Improvement:

 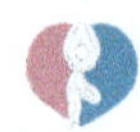

- Cold showers are not just for the brave but also for those seeking a mood boost.

- They stimulate the production of endorphins, the wellness hormones, providing a feeling of joy and reducing stress.

- It's like starting each day on the right foot!

- Cold exposure increases the production of noradrenaline and endorphins.

- These neurotransmitters enhance attention, concentration, and consequently, mood.

- A natural and pleasant way to combat depression and improve your outlook.

3. Strengthening of the Immune System:

- Surprising, right? Cold exposure can stimulate the immune system.

- It increases the production of white blood cells, making your body more resistant to illnesses.

- A natural defense that can make a difference in your overall health.

- Contrary to common beliefs, cold showers boost the immune system.

- The production of lymphocytes, the guardians of your immune system, increases with cold exposure.

- A natural defense against colds and flu.

4. Boosting Metabolism and Fat Burning:

- The magic of thermogenesis is activated with cold showers.

- Your metabolism gets a boost, and potentially, you start burning those stubborn fats.

- An extra help for those looking to lose weight.

5. Improvement in Circulation:

- Cold water is like a masseuse for your arteries.

- It stimulates blood circulation, promoting better oxygen and nutrient supply to your tissues.

- A blessing for cardiovascular health.

6. Increase in Cold Tolerance:

- You will be surprised to discover how much your tolerance to cold can improve.

- A useful benefit, especially during winter, when facing low temperatures will be less unpleasant.

7. Reduction of Inflammation:

 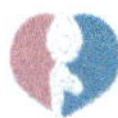

- It fights inflammation, a key to a healthy and long life.

- Chronic inflammation is linked to many diseases, and cold showers seem to lower inflammatory markers.

- A precious defense against degenerative diseases.

8. Development of Mental Strength:

- Facing cold water requires determination.

- This growing practice will make you mentally stronger, better able to handle stress and daily challenges.

- A benefit that goes beyond the physical.

9. Fat Burning and Weight Loss:

- Stimulating brown fat in the body can help you burn accumulated white fat.

- Cold exposure increases metabolism, promoting weight loss.

- An ally for those looking to shape their figure.

10. Improvement in Physical Endurance:

- Mitochondrial biosynthesis is enhanced by cold exposure.

- More mitochondria mean more energy for your cells.

Beyond these tangible benefits, cold showers represent a daily challenge that, over time, will contribute to your mental and physical well-being in surprising ways.

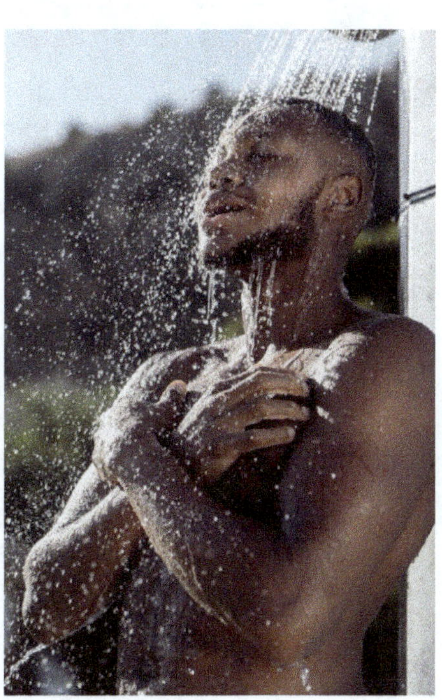

 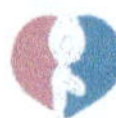

Chapter 4: How to Start a Good Habit

Have you ever looked at your friend and wondered how she manages to stay in shape so effortlessly while you struggle to achieve the same results? And your friend, always impeccable in his work, how does he do it? It's natural to wonder how some people seem to manage their lives so smoothly. The truth is that neither your friend is inherently more attractive, nor your friend is genetically superior. The difference lies in their daily habits. In this chapter, I want to tell you that the difference between an ordinary life and a successful one can often be a small change in your daily habits. You too can transform your life, and often the key is in making small changes in your daily routines.

The Simple Rule for Radical Change

The golden rule we will explore in this chapter is one of the most powerful: make your habits easy, extremely easy. But what does that mean? Who among us has not tried to set big goals at the beginning of the year, only to find themselves giving up shortly after? The key is to make the habit so easy that there is no reason to avoid it.

Have you ever started a project enthusiastically only to give up when it became too demanding?

Let's reflect on an experiment undertaken by a photography professor. Two groups of students, one evaluated on the quality of a single photo and the other on the quantity of photos produced.

A photography professor decided to test this theory. Two groups of students were created: one where the evaluation was based on the quality of a single photo and the other on the quantity of photos produced. Surprisingly, the "quantity" group also produced the highest quality photos. The lesson? Focus on practice and repetition, not initial perfection.

The Two-Minute Rule

The two-minute rule is your key to success. Whatever you want to start, make sure it takes less than two minutes. Don't plan to read a book a day or exercise for two hours every day. Start with one page or one minute of walking. Start small, make the habit simple.

The Importance of Repetitions

 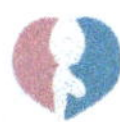

Don't think about the time it will take to develop the habit; think about the repetitions needed. Neuroplasticity shows that the more you repeat an action, the more your brain changes. Never exceed two minutes to make the experience enjoyable. Stop when you feel good. It's the constant practice, not the planning, that changes your brain and creates new habits.

Leave a Good Memory

As Hemingway said, stop when things are going well. Never make the activity so difficult that it deters you. Stop when you are satisfied, and each time it will be easier to repeat the action.

Start with Simplicity

Whether you want to exercise more, eat better, read more, or write a book, start simply. The two-minute rule is your key to changing habits. Be consistent, not perfect. Start now, because small daily habits are the key to lasting change.

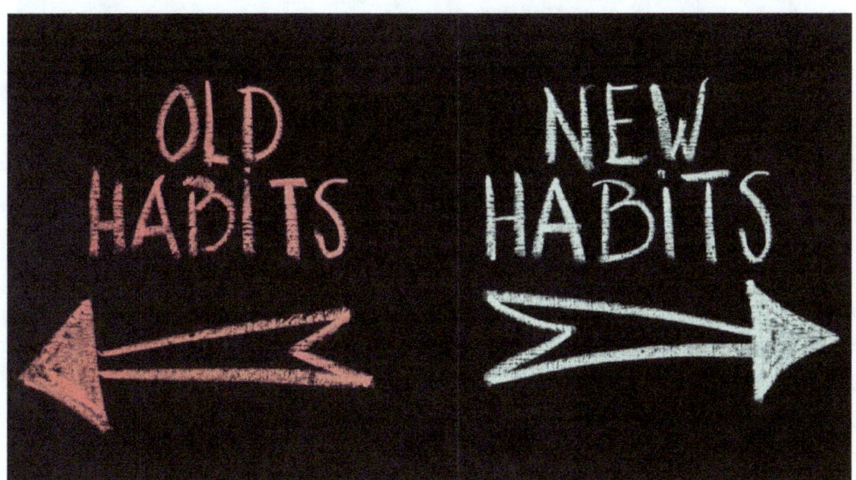

Chapter 5: How to Reduce Inflammation

Have you ever heard that exercise is the key to reducing inflammation? In this chapter, I want to guide you through discovering the true system for improving your health through physical activity.

Exercise isn't just about weight or metabolism. Not at all. Together, we'll uncover the truth about exercise and its impact not only on physical fitness but also on your overall health.

The Myths About Exercise

- Exercise is not just for losing weight or speeding up metabolism. So why is it so essential?

Many people associate exercise exclusively with weight loss or speeding up metabolism. However, the reality is much more multifaceted and rich in benefits beyond simple weight management. In this chapter, we'll debunk some common myths about exercise and discover why it's so essential for your overall well-being.

1. Myth: "Exercise is just for losing weight."

   - Reality: Weight loss is just one of the countless advantages of regular physical activity. Exercise helps improve cardiovascular health, boost the immune system, reduce stress, and enhance mood. Focusing solely on weight loss overlooks a complete range of benefits that physical activity can offer.

2. Myth: "Exercise is just for speeding up metabolism."

   - Reality: While exercise does contribute to metabolism, its impact goes beyond simply increasing calorie burning. Physical activity improves insulin sensitivity, promotes muscle building, and optimizes the overall functioning of your body. Metabolic health is just one of the aspects improved by regular training.

3. Myth: "Exercise is just for the body, not for the mind."

   - Reality: Physical activity has been shown to have a significant impact on mental health. It reduces stress, improves mood, and increases concentration. Exercise releases endorphins, the feel-good hormones, which positively influence emotional and cognitive aspects. Engaging in physical activity is an effective way to improve your mood and mental clarity.

4. Myth: "Exercise is only for athletes or young people."

 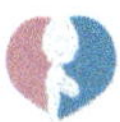

- Reality: Exercise is crucial at all ages. It helps improve physical endurance, flexibility, and strength, which are essential for a healthy and active life. Regular training is associated with greater longevity and a better overall quality of life.

5. Myth: "Only sick people need to exercise."

- Reality: Physical activity is a powerful form of disease prevention. It reduces the risk of cardiovascular diseases, diabetes, osteoporosis, and many other conditions. Regular exercise is a key strategy for maintaining long-term health.

Ultimately, exercise shouldn't be seen as a burdensome task to achieve a specific goal, but as a daily investment in your total health. Beyond aesthetic benefits, physical activity helps build a resilient body and mind. Let exercise become a pillar of your life, a way to celebrate your body and promote your overall well-being.

The Connection Between Exercise and Overall Health

Let's discover the direct links between exercise and your body's inflammation, as well as its influence on steroid hormone levels in your blood.

It's essential to explore the direct connection between physical activity and overall well-being. In this chapter, you'll discover the intricate links between exercise and body inflammation, as well as understanding the influence on the balance of steroid hormones in your system.

1. Reduction of Inflammation:

Inflammation is a natural response of the body to stress or damage. However, chronic inflammation can contribute to many diseases, including heart and metabolic diseases. Regular exercise is a powerful natural anti-inflammatory. During physical activity, the body produces molecules called cytokines, which have anti-inflammatory effects, helping to modulate your body's inflammatory response.

2. Influence on Steroid Hormone Levels:

Steroid hormones, such as cortisol and testosterone, play a crucial role in regulating a range of bodily functions, from energy to metabolism, mood, and sexual health. Exercise has been shown to positively influence these hormones, helping to maintain an optimal balance.

- Cortisol:

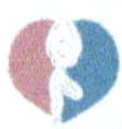

- Moderate exercise helps regulate cortisol levels, also known as the stress hormone. Proper cortisol regulation is essential to avoid negative health effects, such as abdominal fat accumulation and immune system impairment.

- Testosterone:

- Physical activity, especially resistance training, can increase testosterone levels. This is crucial for muscle health, bone density, and even mood. Proper testosterone balance is fundamental to overall well-being.

Thus, exercise is not only a way to stay physically fit but also acts as a global modulator of your biological system. From reducing inflammation to balancing hormones, every session of physical activity acts as a catalyst to optimize your body's functioning.

To maximize the positive effects on inflammation and steroid hormones, try to maintain a regular and varied exercise routine. Include both cardiovascular training and resistance training in your week. Listen to your body and adjust the intensity level based on your individual needs.

In summary, understanding the connection between exercise and overall health is fundamental to shaping a healthy and sustainable lifestyle. Adding physical activity to your daily routine is not only an investment in your physical appearance but also a demonstration of love for your body and mental health.

The Revolutionary Truth

The traditional paradigm of calories burned during exercise has been debunked. It's not just a simple sum of calories but a more complex process. Let's explore the alternative model that can change your approach to physical activity.

If you've always thought of exercise as a simple tool for "burning calories" and counting every sweaty session in terms of energy balance, it's time to embrace a revolutionary truth. The old paradigm of calories burned during exercise has been debunked, and a new way of perceiving physical activity has emerged.

The traditional concept of "calories burned" during exercise is an oversimplification of the complex metabolic process that occurs in your body during physical activity. This traditional model has often led to a quantitative approach, where the amount of exercise is evaluated primarily in terms of calorie balance. However, the reality is much more intricate.

 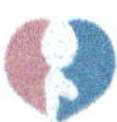

The new paradigm considers exercise as a catalyst for a series of physiological and biochemical processes that go beyond simply "burning calories." Instead of focusing solely on the amount of energy consumed during physical activity, we focus on the long-term impacts on crucial aspects of your health.

Physical activity, particularly moderate-intensity training, can continue to positively influence your metabolism even after you finish exercising. This is known as "post-exercise oxygen consumption" or "afterburn effect." Your body continues to burn calories to restore physiological normalcy.

Regular exercise can lead to improvements in insulin sensitivity and metabolic efficiency. This means your body becomes more adept at using food as a source of energy, positively influencing weight management and metabolic health.

Physical activity can reduce systemic inflammation and positively influence the balance of steroid hormones, with beneficial effects on overall health.

Instead of measuring exercise success solely in terms of "calories lost," embrace a long-term perspective that considers the cascading impacts on your entire biological system. Exercise becomes an investment in your metabolic, hormonal, and general health, bringing positive changes that go far beyond the duration of a single session.

In conclusion, the new exercise paradigm invites you to see physical activity not just as a way to burn calories but as a valuable investment in your overall health. Let your motivation be driven by awareness of the long-term positive impacts, and enjoy the benefits that go far beyond calorie counting.

The Essential Benefits of Exercise

1. Inflammation Control: Exercise reduces the inflammatory response, a key factor in maintaining overall health.

2. Reproductive Hormone Balance: Reproductive hormones are closely linked to cancer risk for both women and men. Exercise helps keep them in check.

"Go exercise!" says the doctor, and there's a reason. Your life could be extended, and diseases could decrease. Let's discover why.

People who exercise have a better cardiovascular system. Let's explore the "6-Minute Walk Test" and its connection to longevity.

 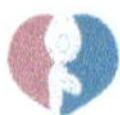

Your heart, the vigorous engine that pumps life through your veins, can reap immense benefits from regular physical activity. Let's explore how exercise helps keep your cardiovascular system in shape, bringing benefits that go beyond mere physical endurance.

When you engage in a regular exercise program, your heart becomes an athlete. Aerobic training, like running, swimming, or cycling, stimulates the heart to pump blood more efficiently. The result is a heart capable of pumping a greater amount of blood with each beat, improving the overall efficiency of the cardiovascular system.

Regular exercise is a powerful ally in managing blood pressure. Physical activity can help keep blood vessels flexible and reduce peripheral resistance, two key factors that influence blood pressure. This is particularly significant for preventing conditions like hypertension.

Physical activity can positively influence cholesterol levels. By reducing LDL ("bad") cholesterol and increasing HDL ("good") cholesterol, exercise helps maintain a balanced lipid profile, reducing the risk of plaque buildup in the arteries.

A practical measure of cardiovascular fitness is the "6-Minute Walk Test." This test evaluates your ability to walk for six minutes at a steady pace. Your performance in this test can provide valuable information about your cardiovascular health and endurance.

The connection between exercise and longevity is evident. People who regularly engage in physical activity have a greater likelihood of living longer lives and, more importantly, enjoying a higher quality of life in old age. Keeping your heart healthy through exercise directly contributes to healthier aging.

High-intensity exercise, such as interval training, can lead to an increase in nitric oxide. This compound promotes the dilation of blood vessels, improving circulation and reducing blood pressure. Additionally, the increase in nitric oxide can have added benefits for vascular health.

Intense activity releases nitric oxide, promoting better vascular health and even improving sexual activity.

Let's now debunk the myth about extreme physical exercise, with the potential negative consequences of extreme exercise, especially for the reproductive and immune systems:

 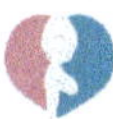

The enthusiasm for physical activity can push us towards extremes that could have negative health consequences. Let's see together how extreme exercise can affect the body, particularly the reproductive and immune systems, debunking some myths that may circulate in this context.

Reproductive System:

- Myth: Extreme Exercise is Only Beneficial.

- Reality: While moderate exercise is generally beneficial for the reproductive system, excess can lead to problems. In women, excessive physical activity can cause menstrual disorders and even amenorrhea, the absence of menstruation. In men, excessive exercise has been associated with a decrease in sperm production.

In conclusion, exercise is a precious gift for your heart. Every step you take, every beat your heart makes during physical activity, contributes to optimal cardiovascular health. Your dedication to exercise not only increases your physical endurance but also the resilience of your heart, preparing it for a longer and healthier life.

2. Oxidative Stress:

- Myth: More Exercise is Always Better.

- Reality: Extreme exercise can trigger excessive oxidative stress. If not managed properly, this stress can damage the body's cells, including those of the reproductive system. A moderate approach to exercise is often healthier.

3. Immune Compromises:

- Myth: Intense Exercise Strengthens Immunity.

- Reality: While moderate exercise can improve immune function, excess can have the opposite effect. Immunity may temporarily decrease after very intense workout sessions, making the body more susceptible to infections. Proper recovery is essential.

4. Overtraining Syndrome:

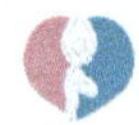

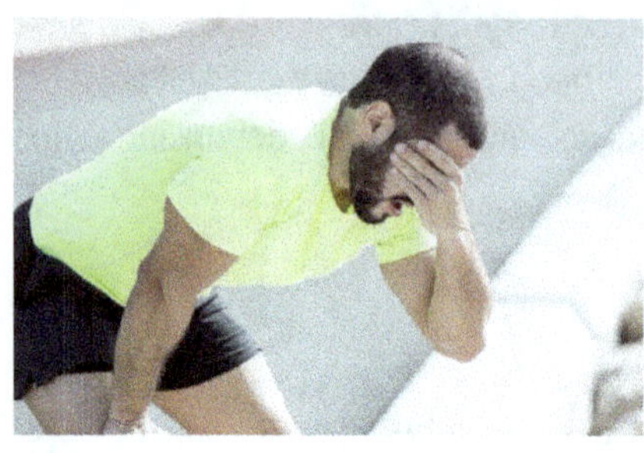

- Myth: Training Every Day is Ideal.

- Reality: Excessive training can lead to a condition known as overtraining syndrome. This condition can result in chronic fatigue, sleep disturbances, and compromised immune function. The importance of rest and variety in training becomes evident.

5. Body Awareness:

- Myth: Ignore Your Body's Signals.

- Reality: A "more is better" approach can lead to ignoring clear signals from the body. Chronic fatigue, persistent pains, and reproductive problems are warning signs that require attention. Listening to your body is crucial.

In conclusion, extreme exercise can carry risks beyond benefits. Seeking a wise balance between physical activity, rest, and listening to your body is essential for maintaining optimal health. Rather than falling into the trap of "more is better," embrace a perspective that values balance and awareness of your body. Your overall health will benefit from this thoughtful and sustainable approach to physical activity.

A New Approach to Weight Loss

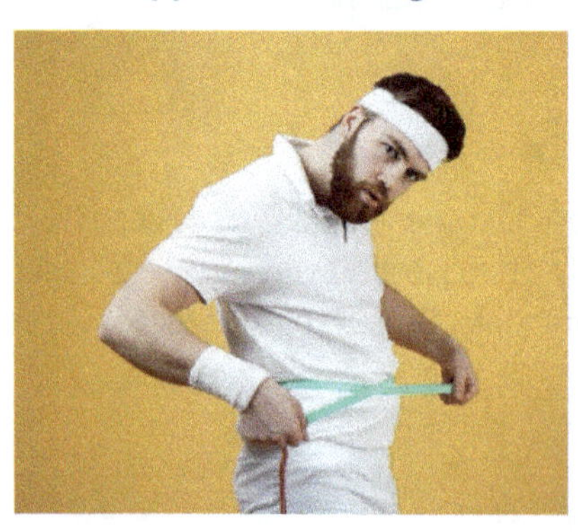

- Discover why exercise is crucial for those trying to lose weight and how it can prevent the yo-yo effect, which often accompanies traditional diets:

Sustainable Weight: A New Approach to Exercise and Weight Loss

Weight loss is often approached through drastic and restrictive diets, but the crucial role of exercise in this journey is often underrated. In this segment, we explore why exercise is fundamental for weight loss and how it can prevent the yo-yo effect associated with traditional diets.

1. Active Metabolism:

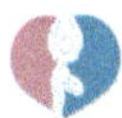

Many diets promise immediate results through extreme calorie restrictions, but this often leads to a slowing down of metabolism, creating a cycle of weight loss and gain.

Exercise helps keep metabolism active, contributing to burning calories consistently even after the workout. This counters the yo-yo effect, supporting more sustainable weight loss.

2. Building Muscle Mass:

Many drastic diets can lead to the loss of muscle mass along with fat, weakening the body and slowing down metabolism.

Resistance training, such as weightlifting, helps preserve and build muscle mass. More muscles mean a more active metabolism and a more toned physique.

3. Combating Stress and Emotional Eating:

Stress and emotions often lead to less healthy food choices. Traditional diets often do not address this psychological component.

Physical activity is a powerful antidote to stress, releasing endorphins that improve mood. This can reduce the impulse to resort to food in response to stress, contributing to healthier weight management.

4. Improving Food Awareness:

Strict Diets and Loss of Control:

Overly restrictive diets can lead to episodes of binge eating when broken, creating a cycle of excessive restriction followed by loss of control.

Exercise can promote greater awareness of the body and its needs. Learning to respond to hunger and satiety signals is crucial for maintaining a healthy weight in the long term.

Sustainable weight loss goes beyond temporary diets. Exercise becomes an essential companion, supporting your metabolic, physical, and mental health. Integrating physical activity into your daily routine will not only help you lose weight but will support you in a long-term wellness journey, avoiding the highs and lows often associated with extreme diets.

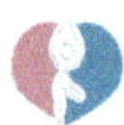

The Paradigm Shift: "Intuitive Eating"

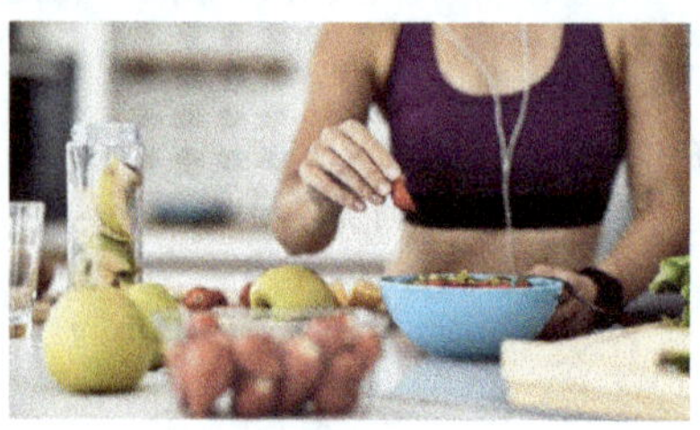

- I introduce you to a revolutionary approach to wellness called "intuitive eating." It's time to consider new ways to approach your health.

Here's a concrete perspective on the importance of exercise for your daily life. I hope this topic inspires you to take a walk, run, or simply move more every day. Your health is a treasure, and exercise is a key to keeping it bright and vibrant:

Intuitive Eating: Listen to Your Body, Nourish Your Soul

Have you ever thought about how often we rely on structured diets without paying attention to our body's signals? Intuitive eating is a revolutionary approach to wellness that promotes food awareness, self-reflection, and a healthier relationship with food. It's time to explore this paradigm shift and understand how it can transform your relationship with food and your health.

1. Listen to Your Body's Signals:

Intuitive eating breaks the chains of restrictive diets. There are no rigid rules, allowing you to respond to your body's needs without guilt.

Listening to natural hunger and satiety signals becomes the compass for your eating. You learn to respect your body, avoiding overeating or neglecting its needs.

2. Awareness as a Guide:

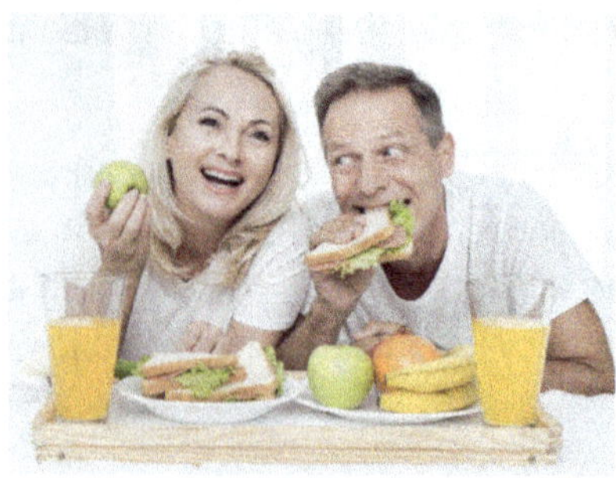

Intuitive eating encourages savoring every bite without distractions. This leads to greater food awareness, helping you recognize flavors and signals from your body.

Food is often tied to emotions. Intuitive eating invites you to explore the connections between food and your emotions, promoting a healthier relationship with food and yourself.

 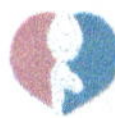

3. No "Good" or "Bad" Food:

The intuitive eating approach eliminates labeling food as "good" or "bad." There are no absolute prohibitions, reducing the forbidden desire that often leads to dysfunctional eating behaviors.

Discover the pleasure of every food without judgment. Intuitive eating encourages enjoying food without guilt, fully embracing the experience without excessive worries about calories or restrictions.

4. A Healthy Relationship with Food:

Intuitive eating frees you from the constant struggle between what you "should" eat and what you "want" to eat. This reduces diet-related stress and improves your relationship with food.

This approach encourages self-compassion. There will be no self-blame or guilt for food choices. You will learn to nourish your body with love and respect.

Intuitive eating is a form of empowerment. It allows you to be the director of your eating, embracing diversity and freedom of choice. This paradigm shift will not only improve your relationship with food but will have a positive impact on your mental and physical health. Try incorporating this approach into your daily life and enjoy the freedom to nourish your body and soul with love and awareness.

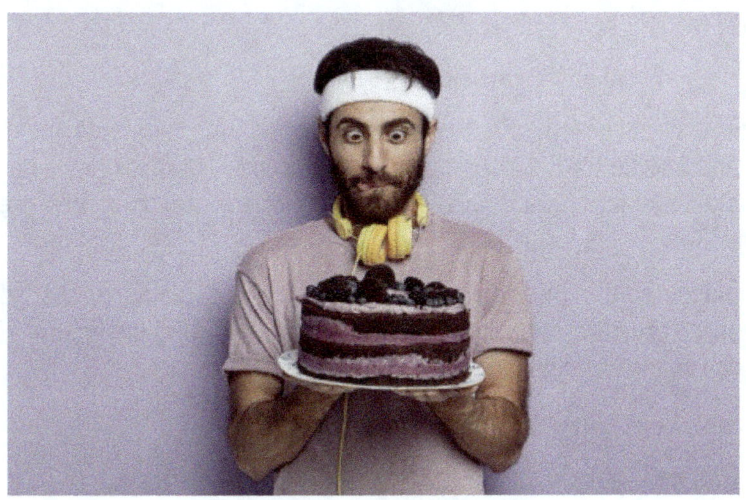

Chapter 6: Discovering the True Reasons behind Weight Loss Difficulty

In the midst of Africa, among the Hadza tribes of northern Tanzania, there's something extraordinary. This was discovered by Herman Pontzer, a paleoanthropologist who traveled the world studying the metabolism of primitive populations and animals. I recently read his book "Burn," which answered many questions and doubts you might also have about the difficulty of losing weight.

Exploring the Habits of the Hadza

- The Hadza, a hunter-gatherer people, live like ancient Prehistoric humans. Pontzer tells us how they risk their lives every day to procure food, even against lions. This underscores how crucial it is for humans to have sufficient nutrients and calories.

The Diet of Primitive Man

- One fundamental question is: what did prehistoric humans eat? Pontzer explores the diet of the Hadza and reveals that humans are opportunistic omnivores, willing to eat anything edible.

Mythical Paleo Diet?

- If you think the Hadza diet is based only on meat, you're mistaken. We discover that their diet mainly consists of carbohydrates from tubers, fruits, plants, insects, and even honey. The reality dispels the myth of the paleolithic diet based solely on animal foods.

The Mystery of Hadza Metabolism

- Pontzer explains how despite the Hadza spending two hours a day in intense activity and walking for 5-6 hours, they only consume 3,000 calories a day, the same as a sedentary Italian. This raises an important question: does exercise really help with weight loss?

It can be deduced that the metabolism model isn't like a steam train that speeds up with more exercise. In reality, our bodies adapt, reducing energy from other areas such as the immune and reproductive systems.

The Crucial Role of the Hypothalamus

The hypothalamus, often referred to as the body's internal clock, plays a crucial role in regulating metabolism. Understanding its function is essential for those seeking to manage body weight in a healthy and sustainable way.

The hypothalamus acts as a sort of central regulator of our metabolism. When you reduce calorie intake or engage in excessive exercise, your body, through the action of the hypothalamus, adapts by lowering basal metabolism. This is an evolutionary adaptation mechanism aimed at preserving energy resources in times of scarcity.

When you follow a low-calorie diet, the hypothalamus detects a decrease in energy reserves and interprets this signal as a potential threat to survival. Consequently, it activates a series of mechanisms to conserve energy. These may include:

- Modulating basal metabolic activity, reducing the number of calories burned at rest.

- Increasing hunger sensation to stimulate energy intake.

- The body may prefer to store fat rather than use it as a primary energy source.

Excessive exercise can also trigger a similar response. If physical activity is extremely intense and prolonged, the hypothalamus may perceive the need to conserve energy, influencing metabolism to adapt to the stress imposed by the workout.

To maintain optimal metabolic well-being, it's crucial to find a balance between calorie intake, physical activity, and your body's individual needs. Some useful approaches include:

- Opt for diets that provide the necessary calories to support your activity level and maintain an active metabolism.

- Practice regular and balanced exercise, avoiding excess that may induce adaptation responses from the hypothalamus.

- Stay mindful of hunger and satiety cues, respecting your body's signals to maintain metabolic balance.

Every individual is unique, and the hypothalamic response can vary from person to person. It's important to adopt a personalized approach that considers your body's specific needs.

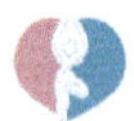

The hypothalamus plays a fundamental role in metabolism management, adapting the body to changes in calorie intake and physical activity. Understanding this mechanism can help you develop more mindful approaches to maintain balanced metabolic health. Listen to your body, respect its needs, and strive to find a sustainable balance to promote your metabolic health.

The Myth of Drastic Diets

- We discover the detrimental effects of extreme diets, such as forced fasting or extreme weight loss TV programs. The hypothalamus reacts like an alarm bell, pushing to regain lost weight.

The Revolutionary Approach: Intuitive Eating

- A revolutionary solution called "intuitive eating" is glimpsed, which we'll explore in detail in an upcoming video. An approach that could radically change how we approach diet and weight loss.

An Appeal to Awareness

- Before concluding, Pontzer emphasizes that exercise may not help with weight loss, but it's vital for overall health. An invitation to understand that movement is essential for multiple aspects of our bodies.

I hope this chapter has provided you with a clearer insight into why many diets and exercise programs may not yield the desired results. Each of us is different, and the key may lie in listening to your body and adopting sustainable habits over time.

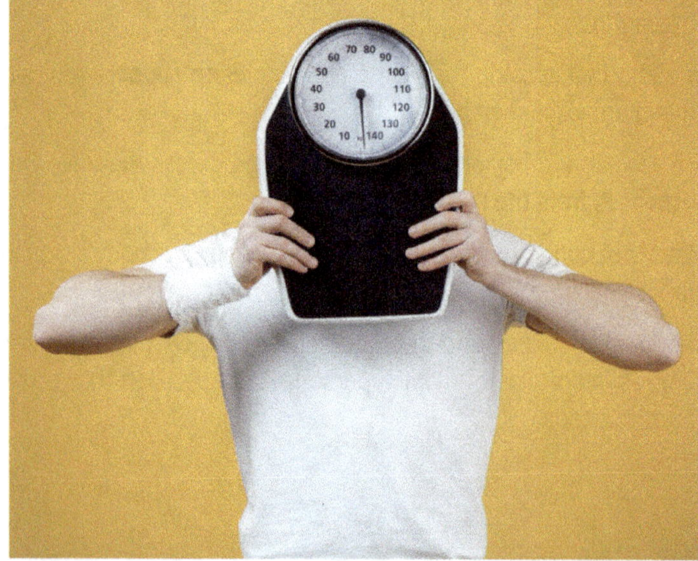

 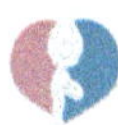

Chapter 7: 6 Natural Anti-inflammatory Foods

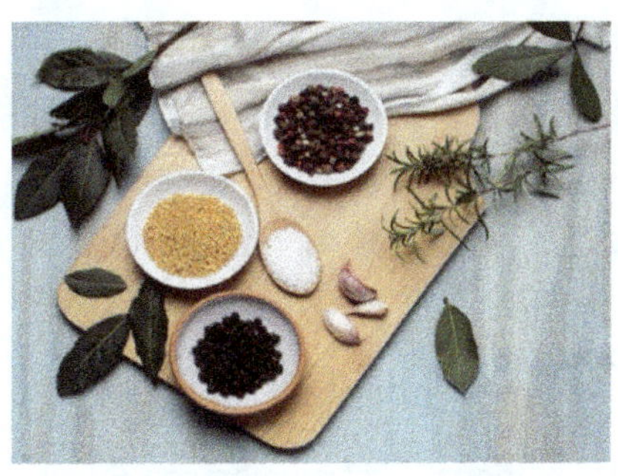

Image from "https://it.freepik.com

I understand how frustrating it can be to deal with daily inflammation in the body, especially when it comes to chronic issues that require long-term use of anti-inflammatory medications. I understand your concerns about the side effects of these medications, and I would like to share with you six powerful natural alternatives. Together, we will explore foods that you can incorporate without restrictions to improve your health, avoiding the undesired side effects of conventional medications.

1. Turmeric:

- Imagine walking through crowded markets in India, where turmeric is valued for its anti-inflammatory properties.

- Turmeric not only reduces inflammation but also offers gastroprotective, liver-protective, and anticancer benefits.

- It stimulates bile production, improving digestion, and protects against gallstone formation.

2. Ginger:

- Another gift from India and China, ginger is the perfect companion to turmeric.

- Besides reducing inflammation, ginger is effective in managing chronic pain, improving mobility, and lowering blood sugar levels.

- It is known to alleviate nausea, muscle pains, and contribute to weight loss.

3. Rosemary:

- Imagine the aromatic scent of rosemary, a plant with remarkable antimicrobial properties.

- Rosemary can be consumed as tea, helping to counteract the proliferation of harmful bacteria in the gut.

 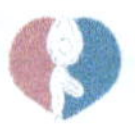

- It is recommended to use concentrated essential oils only under medical advice.

4. Capsaicin (Chili Pepper):

- Capsaicin, found in chili peppers, is not only spicy but also has potent anti-inflammatory and anticancer properties.

- It reduces chronic pain, speeds up metabolism, and helps control appetite.

5. Omega-3 from Algae:

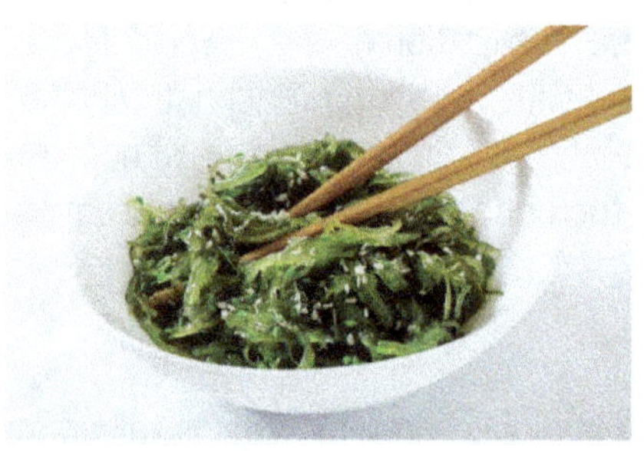

- Break the cycle of high omega-6 levels with a direct source of omega-3: algae.

- Algae provide the primary source of omega-3 found in fish, without the omega-6 imbalance common in Western diets.

6. Green Tea:

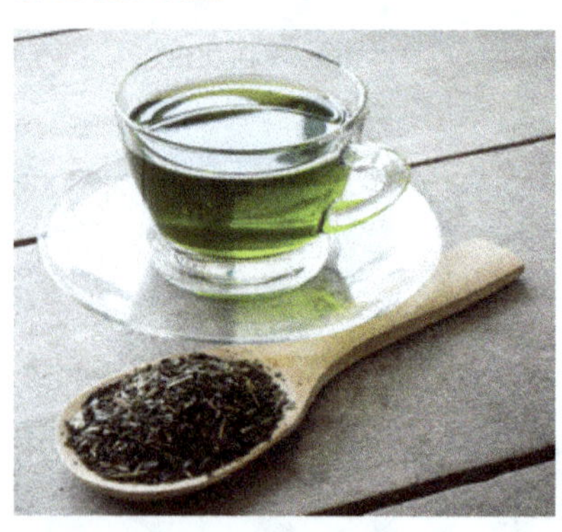

- Picture a tranquil tea ceremony as you discover the benefits of green tea.

- It is recommended during intermittent fasting, preserving the positive effects of fasting on your health.

I understand how difficult it can be to resist frequent use of anti-inflammatory drugs. I want to encourage you to consider these natural options, not only as a short-term solution but as a gradual transformation of your lifestyle. Imagine experiencing the benefits of these foods, not only to fight inflammation but also to improve your overall health. Not only will you be better able to manage pain and inflammation, but you can also reduce reliance on conventional medications, creating a path to long-term wellness. Remember, the power of healing is in your hands.

 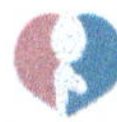

Chapter 8: Most Damaging Foods for the Immune System

Your health and your immune system. In this historical period, it is essential to pay close attention to how we take care of ourselves, especially considering the threat of viruses.

Your primary defense: the immune system

I imagine you are looking for ways to protect yourself from potential threats, and our immune system is the key to doing so. It's like your personal army ready to defend you from pathogens trying to enter your body.

The insidious enemy: oxidative stress

We have done a lot of research to understand how we can strengthen the immune system, and one of the main enemies is oxidative stress. This condition can compromise your health, increase vulnerability to infections, and particularly viruses.

Among all foods, there is one that is particularly harmful to the immune system: fructose. This sugar, found in many processed foods and beverages, has been identified as the main cause of oxidative stress. Now, I don't just want to tell you to stop eating fructose; I want you to understand the reason behind this recommendation.

It inhibits Vitamin D: Fructose inhibits enzymes that convert vitamin D into an active form, compromising your ability to assimilate it correctly.

It inhibits glutathione: This sugar interferes with glutathione, a powerful antioxidant present in cells, compromising your ability to counteract cellular oxidation.

It shields the virus: More insidiously, fructose wraps around the virus like a shield, making it practically invisible to your immune system.

Take a look at your diet:

Now, it's important to examine your diet and make mindful choices. Avoid canned foods, snacks, bread, and sweets, as they are often high in fructose. Look around, you might be surprised where this sugar hides!

Important steps for your health:

1. Intermittent fasting: Science supports intermittent fasting as an effective way to reduce oxidative stress and improve overall health.

 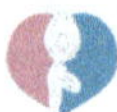

2. Quality sleep: Sleep is essential for reducing oxidative stress and strengthening the immune system. Do not neglect your rest!

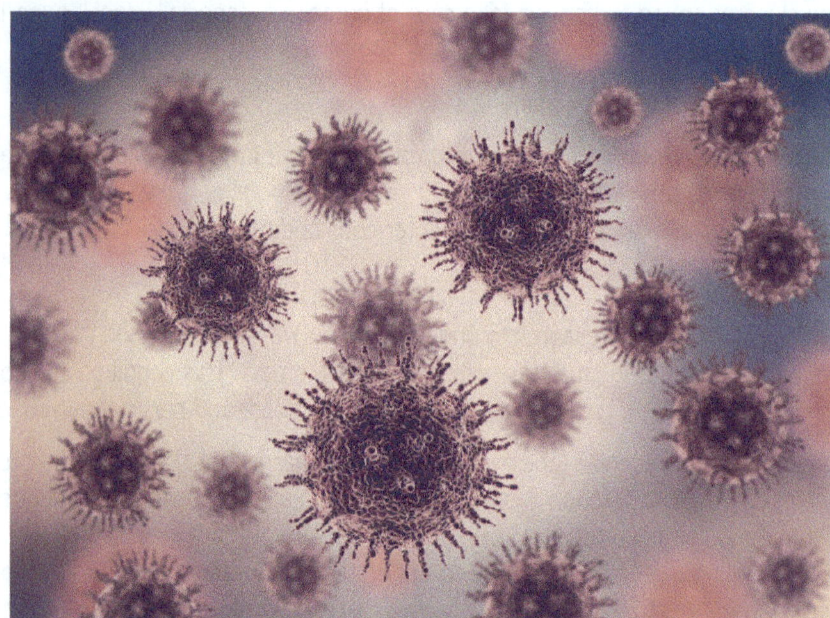

3. Consult experts: If you need specific support for your health, don't hesitate to consult nutritionists, psychologists, and doctors ready to help you.

In conclusion, take care of your body. Your diet plays a fundamental role in your defense against viruses. I hope this information is helpful to you.

 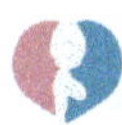

Chapter 9: Ten Foods for Weight Loss and Nurturing Your Well-being

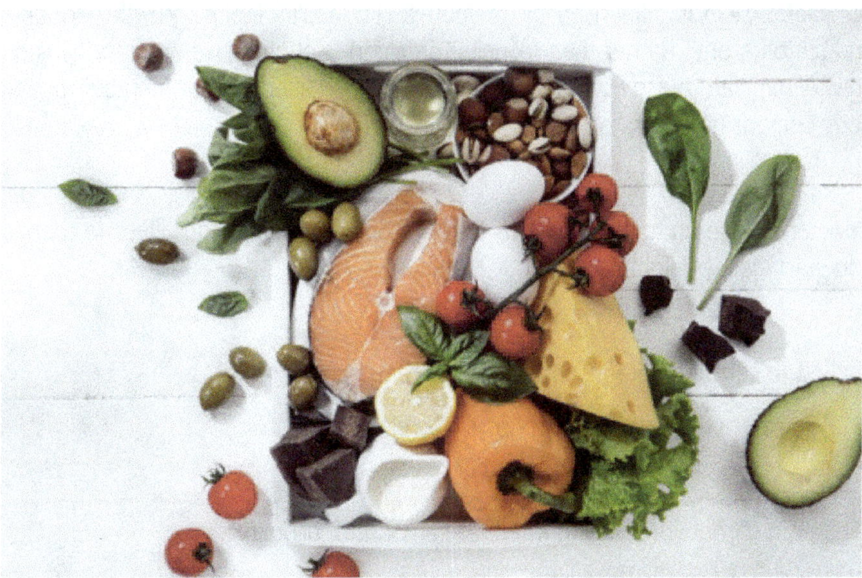

If you've wondered what to eat throughout the day to lose weight consistently and sustainably, you're in the right place. Today, we'll explore together the ten foods that I consider essential for this journey of change. But before we dive into the details, let's reflect for a moment: what is the best way to lose weight? And is it really that important? Let's begin exploring this chapter together:

Why Not Fasting or Extreme Diets?

You may have heard of fasting or extremely low-calorie diets, but are they long-term strategies? Resisting for a day or even for a few days is feasible, but what about long-term? Low-calorie diets often fail because they offer temporary benefits without addressing the necessary lifestyle change. We wouldn't just want to see a few pounds less on the scale, but we want lasting change, right?

The Key is in Lifestyle Change

Losing weight shouldn't mean starving or embarking on draconian diets. It's much more meaningful to start introducing foods that keep us satisfied for longer periods. But you might be wondering, don't calories count? Yes, they do, but science has taught us that it's not just the quantity of calories but how they are managed, assimilated, and burned by our bodies.

 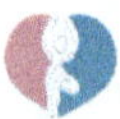

Hormones and Metabolism

Our metabolism is influenced by hormones like insulin, leptin, growth hormone, and testosterone. Rather than focusing on calorie counting, we need to focus on how to stimulate these hormones to have a positive effect on our metabolism and body composition.

The 10 Key Foods for Change

Now, let's move on to the ten foods that I recommend to kickstart lifestyle change and start losing weight.

1. Coconut Cream:

- Low in carbohydrates, sugars, and proteins.

- Rich in healthy fats that keep insulin levels low.

2. Yogurt and Cheese:

- Low in carbohydrates and moderate amount of protein.

- Watch out for lactose intolerances; opt for aged cheeses and homemade yogurt.

3. Sardines and Fatty Fish:

- Rich in omega-3, essential for cellular health.

- Zero carbohydrates and less mercury exposure compared to large fish.

4. Olive Oil and Coconut Oil:

- Zero carbohydrates, rich in healthy fatty acids.

- Help keep blood sugar and insulin low.

5. Nuts:

- Walnuts, almonds, Macadamia.

- Rich in healthy fats and fiber that increase satiety.

6. Leafy Greens and Cruciferous Vegetables:

- Essential carbohydrates, rich in vitamins and minerals.

- Important for health and feeling of fullness.

 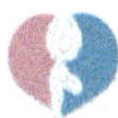

7. Avocado:

- Rich in healthy fatty acids, beneficial for hormones like testosterone and leptin.

8. Eggs:

- Considered nutrient-dense and healthy despite old myths.

- Prefer eggs from free-range chickens.

9. Chicken Thighs:

- Pay attention to chicken feed.

- Prefer meat from reliable and naturally raised sources.

10. Fatty Meat (Optional):

- Include once a week or every two weeks.

- Also eat the fatty part, it brings significant benefits.

These foods, suitable for vegans, vegetarians, omnivores, and carnivores, can be the key to stimulating the right hormones, improving your metabolism, and helping you lose weight. Prepare them carefully, enjoy them fully, and observe the positive changes in your body and health. It's not just about losing weight, but becoming a healthier person in tune with your body.

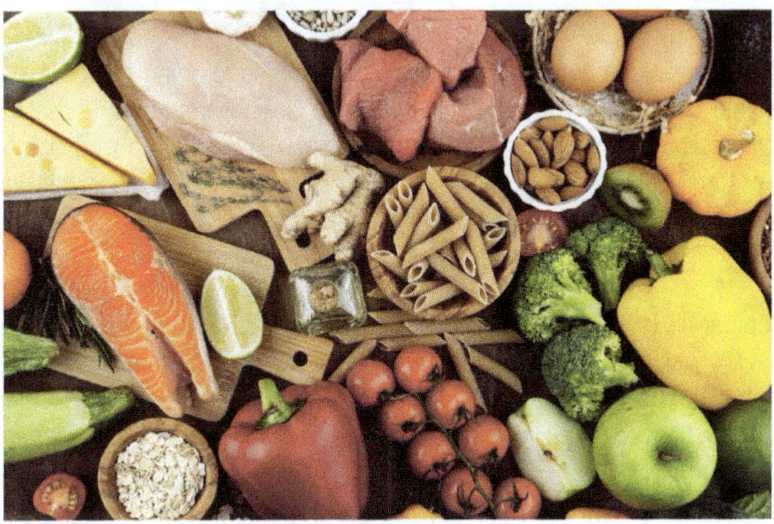

Chapter 10: How to Detoxify Your Body from Pesticides

We've made a discovery that could make a difference to your well-being and health. In this chapter, we'll explore in-depth how to rid your body of pesticides, harmful agents that can sneak into your daily life in unsuspected ways. It will be a journey of genuine love for your body, full of practical advice and vital information to restore your well-being.

Among the wide range of factors influencing the slowdown of metabolism, one of the main culprits seems to be pesticides. Not only do they make weight loss difficult for those who are overweight, but they also seem to contribute to how easily people of normal weight can gain weight. Together, we'll explore practical strategies to reduce pesticide levels in your body, allowing you to restore a healthy metabolism.

Pesticides are everywhere, from the products you eat to the surfaces you come into contact with. We'll start this exploration by understanding the scope of this daily exposure and how pesticides can accumulate in your body over time.

Listen to Your Body: Warning Signs of Pesticides

Your body is wise and often communicates when something is wrong. We'll discuss the signs that might indicate the presence of pesticides in your body, from skin irritations to chronic fatigue. You'll learn to listen carefully to your body to understand when it's time to take action:

One crucial aspect of your battle against pesticides is learning to decipher the signals your body sends you. Whether you realize it or not, your body is constantly in communication with you, and understanding warning signs can be crucial to intervene promptly against pesticide presence. Here are some signs that might indicate the presence of these harmful substances in your body:

1. Skin Irritations and Dermatological Problems:

The epidermis is the body's largest organ and can act as a barrier against pesticides. However, skin irritations, redness, or rashes could be signs of exposure to harmful chemicals. Pay attention to sudden changes in your skin and allergic reactions, as they could be your body's way of asking for help.

2. Persistent Fatigue and Chronic Tiredness:

 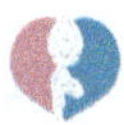

Persistent tiredness and lack of energy could result from an overload of pesticides in your system. These chemicals can affect your metabolism and your body's ability to convert food into energy. If you experience constant fatigue despite adequate rest, it might be time to carefully examine your pesticide exposure.

3. Gastrointestinal Disturbances:

Pesticides can negatively affect the health of your digestive tract. Issues like bloating, abdominal cramps, or irregular bowel movements could be signs of an excessive presence of unwanted chemicals in your body. Monitor your digestive habits closely to detect any changes.

4. Changes in Cognitive Function:

Some pesticides can influence brain function and your ability to concentrate. If you've noticed memory difficulties, confusion, or concentration problems that seem inexplicable, it might be worth examining your pesticide exposure and trying to reduce it.

5. Respiratory Symptoms:

Pesticide exposure can also affect the respiratory system, causing symptoms like persistent cough, difficulty breathing, or irritation of the respiratory tract. If you experience these symptoms without an apparent cause, it could be linked to the environment around you.

Learning to recognize these signals is an act of self-love. Listening carefully to your body not only allows you to identify potential threats to your health but also gives you the power to act proactively. When you notice these signals, don't ignore them. Start a dialogue with your body, try to identify the sources of exposure, and take steps to reduce it.

Remember that you are the guardian of your well-being, and listening to your body is a significant step toward a healthier and more conscious lifestyle. Are you ready to listen and respond to your body's message?

The Power of Detox: From Food to Herbs

Let's explore the fundamental role of food as a defense against pesticides. You'll learn about nutrient-rich foods that support the detoxification process and discover how some herbs can be valuable allies in cleansing your body:

1. Detoxifying Foods:

Food is more than just fuel; it can be your weapon against pesticides. Some foods are particularly effective in supporting your body's detoxification process. Incorporate them into your diet to boost your health:

- Organic Fruits and Vegetables: Choosing organic products reduces pesticide exposure. Fresh fruits and vegetables, especially those high in fiber like apples, kiwi, cabbage, and spinach, are rich in antioxidants that support detoxification.

- Garlic and Onion: These foods not only add flavor to your dishes but also contain compounds that support the liver, the main organ involved in detoxification.

- Turmeric: With its anti-inflammatory and antioxidant properties, turmeric can play a key role in protecting the body from pesticide damage. Add it to your recipes to enjoy its benefits.

- Cucumber: With its high water content, cucumber helps hydrate the body and supports kidney function, thus aiding in the toxin elimination process.

2. Detoxifying Herbs:

Herbs have a long history of use in traditional medicine to improve health and support detoxification. Add these herbs to your arsenal to strengthen your defense system:

Artichoke:

- Promotes bile production, supporting the liver in removing toxic substances from the body.

Milk Thistle:

- Known for its protective properties on the liver, milk thistle can be a valuable ally in your detoxification journey.

Parsley:

- Rich in vitamins and minerals, parsley has diuretic properties that can help eliminate toxins through urine.

Ginger:

 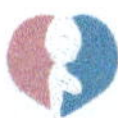

- Its anti-inflammatory properties can support your immune system while working to eliminate unwanted substances.

Choosing an Organic Diet:

- Opt for foods from organic farming.

- Studies show a significant reduction in pesticide levels in the urine of those who follow organic farming practices.

- The diet should focus on plants, vegetables, fruits, whole grains, and legumes, rich in essential fiber for intestinal cleansing.

Limiting the Consumption of Fish and Dairy:

- Reduce the intake of fish, especially those large in size and naturally fatty, known for accumulating pesticides.

- Dairy products such as milk and cheese can also be rich in pesticides due to animal feeding.

Your diet and the use of herbs can play a crucial role in your fight against pesticides. Choose nutritious foods and integrate beneficial herbs to support your body's natural detoxification process. Remember, investing in your health through conscious food choices is an act of love towards yourself and your long-term well-being.

Hydration as the Key to Success

Water is life, and in our case, it is also a powerful detoxification tool. I will guide you through optimal hydration methods to help your body eliminate pesticides naturally.

Water as a Detox Elixir: Optimal Hydration for Eliminating Pesticides

1. The Importance of Hydration:

Water is much more than just a refreshing drink; it is a vital elixir for your health. In the context of detoxifying from pesticides, hydration plays a crucial role in supporting the body in eliminating unwanted substances. Here's how you can optimize your water intake for an effective detoxification process:

2. Adequate Water Quantity:

Ensure you drink enough water every day. The necessary amount can vary depending on your weight, lifestyle, and climate. Generally, aim for an intake of at least 8 glasses of water a day. The goal is to keep your body well-hydrated to promote the natural processes of toxin elimination.

3. Lemon in Water:

Adding lemon juice to your water can offer additional benefits. Lemon is known for its alkalizing properties and can support digestive function. An alkaline environment in your body can promote detoxification and neutralize acidity.

4. Detox Teas:

Consider including herbal detox teas in your daily routine. Teas such as mint, fennel, or dandelion are known for their diuretic properties and can contribute to the elimination of toxins through urine.

5. Hydrating Foods:

Remember that not only water is essential for hydration. Some foods have a high water content and can contribute to your daily liquid intake. Cucumbers, watermelons, melons, and oranges are just a few examples of water-rich foods you can include in your diet.

6. Hydration and Kidney Function:

Water is a key element in supporting kidney function, which plays a crucial role in detoxification. Ensure you drink enough to facilitate the elimination of toxins through urine. Proper kidney function is essential for maintaining balanced fluid levels and ensuring effective system cleansing.

7. Listen to Your Body:

Every individual is unique, and hydration needs can vary. Listen to your body. If you feel thirsty, respond to that sensation. Keeping a water bottle handy throughout the day can serve as a constant reminder to stay hydrated.

Water is a powerful tool in your fight against pesticides. Incorporate these hydration practices into your daily routine and watch how your body responds positively. With adequate water support, you can maximize your body's natural ability to eliminate toxins and promote a healthier internal environment. Remember, every sip is a step towards a cleaner and detoxified life!

The Importance of Physical Exercise

Sweat is one of the most underrated allies in your fight against pesticides. I will share with you how physical exercise not only improves your general health but also serves as a vehicle for expelling accumulated toxins:

Sweat and Movement: Physical Exercise as a Natural Detox

1. Sweat as an Emissary of Toxins:

Sweat is much more than a bodily response to heat. It is a powerful vehicle for expelling accumulated toxins from your body. When you engage in physical activity, your body responds by producing sweat, a mixture of water, salts, and, surprisingly, toxic substances. This natural process is one of the keys to freeing your body from accumulations of pesticides and other unwanted substances.

2. Improvement of Circulation and Detoxification:

Physical exercise, whether it is jogging, swimming, or a yoga session, improves blood circulation. Better circulation means your body can more efficiently transport blood, carrying toxins to elimination organs such as the kidneys and liver. This process is fundamental for detoxification.

3. Exercise to Activate the Lymphatic System:

The lymphatic system plays a crucial role in removing toxins from the body. Physical activity, especially exercises that involve muscle movement, stimulates the lymphatic system. This helps eliminate cellular waste and toxins, contributing to the internal cleansing process.

4. Exercises That Promote Sweating:

Not all exercises generate the same amount of sweat. More intense activities, such as high-intensity interval training (HIIT), running, or saunas, can stimulate greater sweat production. This sweat, rich in toxins, serves as a powerful expulsion vehicle.

5. Sweating to Eliminate Heavy Metals:

In addition to pesticides, sweat is an effective means of eliminating heavy metals. These elements, which can be harmful to health if accumulated in the body, are released through sweat during physical activity.

 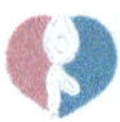

6. Consistency in Exercise:

The key is consistency. It is not necessary to engage in extremely intense workouts every day. Even moderate and regular physical activity has the potential to significantly improve your detoxification process.

Physical exercise is not just about physical fitness but also about internal well-being. Sweat is your secret ally in the fight against pesticides and other harmful substances. Regularly incorporate physical activity into your routine, choosing exercises that promote sweating, and allow your body to rid itself of toxins. Movement is a natural way to improve your health and promote a clean and regenerated internal environment.

Rejuvenating Rest

Sleep is a crucial time when your body repairs and detoxifies itself. We will delve into practices that enhance sleep quality and promote a more effective detoxification process:

Sleep is not just a period of rest, but also a valuable opportunity for your body to perform repair and detoxification processes. We will explore practices that improve sleep quality, making this crucial moment a powerful ally in your detox journey.

1. Deep Sleep and Cellular Repair:

During deep sleep, your body increases the production of growth hormone, necessary for cell repair and muscle growth. This process is fundamental for replacing damaged cells, including those that may have accumulated toxins.

2. The Role of Sleep in Brain Detoxification:

During sleep, the brain's glymphatic system is particularly active. This system acts as the brain's cleaning system, removing toxic waste accumulated during daily activities. Quality sleep is essential to ensure this process occurs effectively.

3. Practices to Improve Sleep Quality:

 - Sleep Routine: Establishing a regular sleep routine by going to bed and waking up at the same time every day helps synchronize your circadian rhythm, improving sleep quality.

 - Optimal Environment: Keeping the bedroom cool, dark, and quiet helps create an environment conducive to deep sleep.

 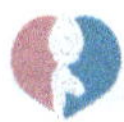

- Limit Blue Light: Reducing exposure to blue light from electronic devices before bedtime can promote the production of melatonin, the sleep hormone.

- Avoid Stimulants: Limiting caffeine and other stimulants intake in the hours leading up to sleep can improve the quality of nighttime rest.

4. Sleep and Hormonal Regulation:

Sleep affects hormonal balance, including hormones involved in hunger and satiety processes. Good sleep quality can help regulate appetite and prevent unhealthy food choices.

5. Meditation for Rejuvenating Sleep:

Practicing meditation before bed can calm the mind, reduce stress, and facilitate a smoother transition to sleep. This approach can significantly improve the quality of your nighttime rest.

Sleep is a powerful ally in your daily fight against toxins. Enhancing sleep quality through mindful practices not only improves your overall well-being but also boosts your body's natural detoxification process. Prioritize quality sleep, and your body will reward you with energy, vitality, and better resistance to harmful substances.

Choose a Conscious Lifestyle

Awareness of your daily choices is a powerful weapon against continuous exposure to pesticides. From choosing personal care products to organic foods, we will explore how daily decisions can make a big difference.

Your daily life is full of choices, and every decision can be an important step towards reducing pesticide exposure. From personal care to choosing organic foods, we will explore how your daily decisions can make a big difference in your fight against pesticides.

1. Toxin-Free Personal Care:

Start with your personal care routine. Many lotions, shampoos, and cosmetics contain harmful chemicals. Switch to natural-based products, preferably certified organic, to reduce the absorption of unwanted chemicals through your skin.

2. Organic Food:

 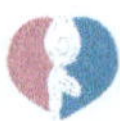

Food choice is a crucial aspect of your exposure to pesticides. Choosing organic food significantly reduces the risk of ingesting pesticide residues. Organic foods are grown without synthetic pesticides, herbicides, or chemical fertilizers.

3. Green Cleaning:

Household cleaning products can be rich in harmful chemicals. Opt for green cleaning products or make your own cleaners using natural ingredients like vinegar, baking soda, and essential oils. This choice not only protects you and your family but also helps reduce environmental impact.

4. Natural Clothing:

Synthetic fabrics may contain traces of pesticides used during the fiber growing process. Choose clothing made from natural materials such as organic cotton, linen, or hemp to reduce contact with harmful chemicals.

5. Natural Gardening:

If you grow your own food or maintain a garden, adopt natural gardening practices. Avoid using chemical pesticides and synthetic fertilizers, opting for organic alternatives. This will not only protect your body but also help preserve the surrounding ecosystem.

6. Label Awareness:

Learn to carefully read product labels. Whether it's food, personal care products, or cleaners, a thorough understanding of labels will help you identify and avoid harmful chemicals.

7. Sharing Awareness:

Awareness is contagious. Share your conscious choices with friends and family. Spreading awareness creates a demand for safer products, encouraging companies to adopt sustainable practices.

Your daily decisions can make a big difference in your pesticide exposure. By choosing natural products, organic foods, and adopting sustainable practices, you are not only protecting your health but also helping to create a safer environment for everyone. Every small choice counts, and together we can make significant strides toward a healthier and more sustainable lifestyle.

 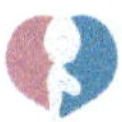

Trust in Nature: Supplements and Natural Remedies

We will delve into the world of supplements and natural remedies that can support your body during the detoxification process. From spirulina to essential oils, discover how nature provides powerful tools for your well-being.

In this section, we will explore the potential of natural remedies and supplements that nature offers to support your body in the detoxification process. From spirulina to essential oils, discover how these powerful tools can contribute to your overall well-being.

1. Spirulina: A Super Detox Supplement:

Spirulina is a nutrient-rich microorganism that grows in fresh water. It is known for its detoxifying properties due to its ability to bind and remove heavy metals from the body. Incorporating spirulina into your daily diet can provide valuable support during the detoxification process.

2. Turmeric: Anti-Inflammatory Properties:

Turmeric is a powerful antioxidant with strong anti-inflammatory properties. Its active ingredient, curcumin, is known to support liver function and reduce inflammation in the body. Add turmeric to your culinary preparations or consider taking supplements to maximize its benefits.

3. Cilantro or Coriander: Removes Heavy Metals:

Cilantro, also known as coriander, is famous for its ability to bind and remove heavy metals such as mercury and lead from the body. You can add fresh cilantro to your salads or blend it into your detox smoothies to harness its purifying properties.

4. Detox Essential Oils:

Essential oils have been shown to have multiple health benefits, including the ability to support detoxification. Oils like lemon, peppermint, and ginger can be used to improve digestion, stimulate the lymphatic system, and promote mental clarity.

5. Chlorophyll: Internal Cleansing:

Chlorophyll-rich foods, such as barley and wheatgrass, are known for their detoxifying properties. Chlorophyll supports internal cleansing, promoting the detoxification of cells and tissues. Consider incorporating chlorophyll-based superfoods into your daily diet.

6. Milk Thistle: Liver Support:

Milk thistle is widely used to support liver health. This herb contains silybin, a compound that has been shown to protect the liver from toxins. Milk thistle supplements can be beneficial for optimizing liver function during detoxification.

7. Bach Flowers: Emotional Balance:

Detoxification is not only about the physical body but also emotional balance. Bach flower remedies offer support for emotional well-being, helping to manage stress, anxiety, and emotions related to the detoxification process.

Relying on nature for supplements and natural remedies is a wonderful way to support your body in the detoxification process. By wisely choosing the right foods and supplements, you can boost your health in a harmonious and natural way. Always remember to consult a health professional before making significant changes to your diet or starting new supplements. Your natural healing journey is a step towards a healthier and more balanced life.

Monitoring and Sustaining Detox

The detoxification process does not end when you start seeing initial results. I will share strategies for constantly monitoring your pesticide exposure and maintaining a mindful approach for a cleaner and more resilient body.

Stop Smoking and Reduce the Use of Chemical Pesticides:

- Smoking contains toxic substances and harmful pesticides, so quitting smoking is a crucial choice for your health.

- Prefer natural remedies like baking soda and vinegar to combat insects or care for your plants, avoiding chemical pesticides.

Donate Blood:

- Blood donation has shown a reduction in the levels of some toxic substances in the body, including pesticides.

- Besides the altruistic benefit, donating blood also offers regular health check-ups through periodic tests.

 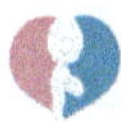

Choosing organic farming, modifying your dietary and daily life habits, and even donating blood are concrete steps you can take to reduce pesticide levels in your body. These actions will not only promote your physical well-being but also have a positive impact on your ability to lose weight healthily and sustainably. Remember, taking care of yourself is an act of self-love.

I encourage you to view your fight against pesticides as a new beginning. It will be an invitation to maintain a conscious lifestyle, with a constant focus on the health and well-being of your body.

Thank you for embarking on this journey with me. Your health is a treasure, and freeing your body from pesticides is an act of love and respect for yourself. May this chapter guide you towards a cleaner and rejuvenated life.

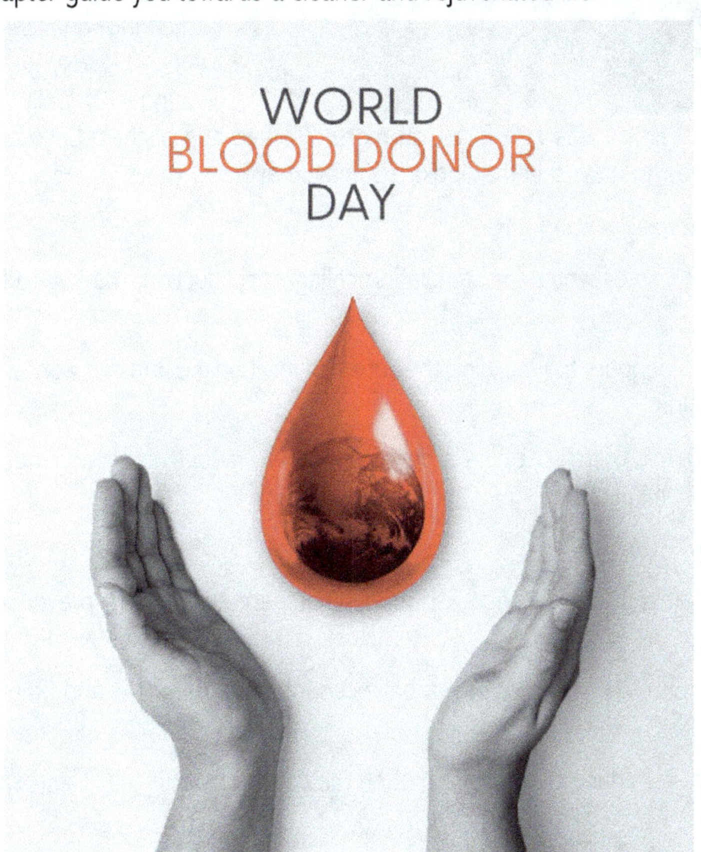

 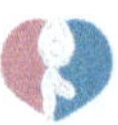

Chapter 11: Secrets for Youthful and Radiant Skin

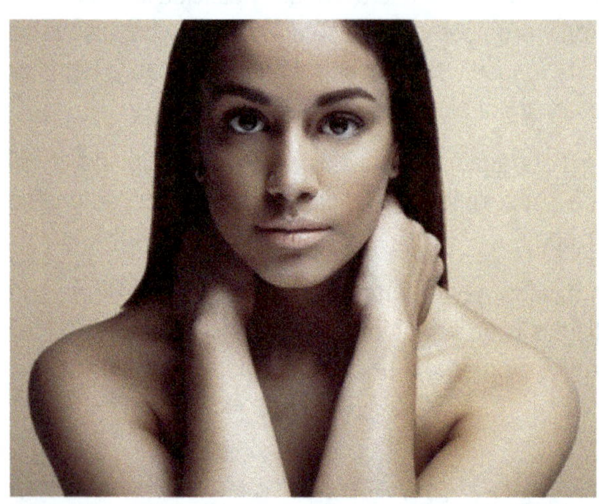

[Image by Anastasia Kazakova on Freepik]

In this chapter, I want to share with you some secrets for achieving younger and more radiant skin. Have you ever thought, inspired by random chit-chat, about smearing guacamole on your face to look younger? Well, forget those funny little ideas and focus on more effective approaches. Let's discover together how to have skin that looks 10, maybe even 20 years younger.

1. Vitamin C and Bell Peppers:

- Vitamin C is essential for stimulating collagen production, the key to healthy skin.

- Add bell peppers to your diet; they are rich in vitamin C and can work wonders for your skin.

- Just 50-75g of bell peppers a day is enough to meet the recommended daily intake of vitamin C.

2. Healthy Fats and Nuts:

- Healthy fats, like the omega-3s found in nuts, are essential for preventing skin aging.

- Eat 2-3 nuts a day to ensure a balanced intake of omega-3 and omega-6 in your diet.

- Omega-3s reduce inflammation, often the cause of skin issues like rosacea or dermatitis.

3. Vitamin A and Cauliflower:

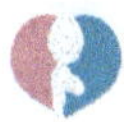

- Cauliflower, rich in vitamins A and C, is a must for a diet that promotes collagen production.

- Vitamin A is crucial for your hormonal balance, important for maintaining healthy, youthful skin.

- Also consume other foods rich in vitamin A, such as eggs and fish.

4. Vitamin E and Sunflower Seeds:

- Vitamin E is fundamental for skin repair and healing.

- Sunflower seeds are a fantastic source of vitamin E and can be easily added to salads or breakfasts.

- Maintain a balance between omega-3 and omega-6 to counteract skin inflammation.

Additional Tips for Healthy Skin:

- Protect Your Skin from the Sun:

  - Excessive sun exposure is the leading cause of skin cancers.

  - Gradually expose yourself to the sun throughout the year to prepare your skin.

  - Use sunscreen to protect yourself, but avoid staying in the sun for too long.

- Avoid Advanced Glycation End Products:

  - Reduce excess sugars, which can contribute to skin problems.

  - Foods processed through advanced glycation can affect your skin.

- Correct Internal Imbalance:

  - Many skin problems are manifestations of an internal issue.

  - Correct hormonal dysfunctions, inflammations, or nutritional deficiencies to benefit both internally and externally.

Remember, your skin is a reflection of your internal health. Take care of yourself by following a balanced diet and adopting a healthy lifestyle. You'll see the results on your skin and feel the benefits throughout your body. Continue following these tips, and your skin will thank you.

 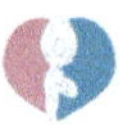

Chapter 12: Seven Strategies to Preserve Your Brain Health

We will tackle a fundamentally important topic together: brain health, especially for women. Yes, you heard that right. Our brain, so complex and wonderful, requires particular attention, and we can no longer ignore the fact that much medical research has primarily focused on men, neglecting the crucial differences involving women's bodies and brains.

Have you ever wondered why the symptoms of a heart attack or the risks related to heart problems are so different between men and women? It's the same when it comes to drug studies, where recommended doses often prove unsuitable or even harmful for women. But today, I want to talk to you about something deeper and more personal: the significantly higher risk that women have of developing dementia and Alzheimer's compared to men. And the main cause? Hormonal dysfunction.

That's why it's so important to understand what a woman can do, both after menopause and before, to preserve her brain and reduce the risk of dementia. Lisa Mosconi, an Italian researcher who has dedicated twenty years to studying the female brain, will guide us through seven practical and fundamental strategies.

Recognize Your Uniqueness

The physiology and biology of women are unique, and ignoring these differences has real consequences on their health. Symptoms like hot flashes, dizziness, and memory loss during menopause are not just "typical" but have a physical and genetic basis within the brain.

The first crucial step towards female well-being is to recognize and value the unique physiology of women. Ignoring these differences can have significant impacts on health, especially during critical phases like menopause. Let's delve into how understanding and respecting your uniqueness can lead to better health management.

Women go through various stages in their lives, each characterized by distinct physiological changes. Ignoring these nuances can lead to a superficial understanding of women's symptoms and specific needs. For example, during menopause, symptoms like hot flashes, dizziness, and memory loss are not just "typical" inconveniences but are rooted in the physiology and genetics of the female brain.

 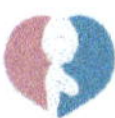

Menopause should not be reduced to a generic stereotype. Each woman experiences this phase uniquely. Understanding your individual experience requires a more in-depth and respectful analysis of your biology. Hot flashes and other symptoms can vary in intensity and duration, and recognizing their complexity is the first step towards conscious management.

Your physiology involves not just the body but also mental health. Women can face specific challenges related to hormonal changes. For instance, variations in estrogen levels can affect mood and mental health. Recognizing this connection is essential for comprehensive well-being management.

It's vital to rely on scientific research and individual awareness. Educating yourself on how your body works, especially in different life stages, empowers you to take targeted care of yourself. Rely on reliable sources and seek support from health professionals specializing in female physiology.

Ultimately, recognizing your uniqueness as a woman is an act of power. Challenge stereotypes, embrace the complexity of your physiology, and strive to understand how each phase of female life is unique. Health is a personal journey, and when you approach it with awareness and respect for your uniqueness, you become the champion of your health.

Hormonal Changes

During puberty and menopause, the female brain undergoes significant hormonal changes that directly influence brain development. Female hormones, such as estrogen, play a crucial protective role for the brain.

Puberty marks the beginning of an extraordinary journey for every woman. During this period, the female brain undergoes substantial hormonal changes, an intricate choreography that prepares the body and mind for adulthood. Hormones, primarily driven by estrogen, are key players in this crucial phase of development.

The female brain is an evolving canvas during puberty. Estrogen, besides orchestrating physical development, plays a key role in modulating brain synapses and forming new neural connections. This phase is a moment of neurological adaptation, preparing the woman for the challenges and joys of adulthood.

Estrogen is not only a major player during puberty but continues to perform a crucial protective role for the female brain throughout life. These hormones

 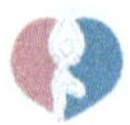

positively influence brain health, providing natural protection against neurodegenerative problems. Their presence helps maintain memory, concentration, and cognitive function.

Menopause, although marked by the end of the menstrual cycle, represents another significant chapter in a woman's journey. During this period, the brain experiences a drastic variation in levels of reproductive hormones, particularly estrogen and progesterone.

The decline in estrogen during menopause can lead to cognitive challenges. Many women report changes in memory and concentration. Understanding these impacts is essential for consciously addressing the challenges that may arise during this phase.

Recognizing the importance of estrogen for brain health is the first step toward conscious management of menopause. A balanced diet, a healthy lifestyle, and, if necessary, medical support can help mitigate the effects of hormonal changes and preserve brain health.

Puberty and menopause are two key chapters in the extraordinary journey of femininity, guided by delicate hormonal changes that directly influence brain health. Promoting an open dialogue about brain health during these phases not only provides awareness but also the possibility of adopting targeted approaches to preserve and enhance the strength and vitality of the female brain.

Make Exercise a Lifelong Companion

Study after study links physical exercise to good cognitive health and reduced risk of dementia. Light or moderate-intensity exercise is particularly beneficial for women, helping to keep the brain active and healthy.

The connection between physical exercise and cognitive health is a symphony of positive results, highlighted by one study after another. Women who incorporate physical activity into their daily routine not only experience improvements in overall health but also enjoy significant cognitive benefits.

Physical exercise, particularly of light or moderate intensity, emerges as a powerful weapon in the fight against dementia. Studies show that women who maintain an active lifestyle have a reduced risk of developing degenerative cognitive

 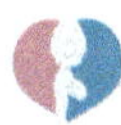

conditions. Physical activity thus becomes a reliable companion in preserving mental clarity and memory.

The intensity of exercise is key, and the wellness ballet of cognitive health requires measured movements. Activities such as walking, swimming, or moderate-intensity yoga become ideal partners for keeping the brain active. This ballet of movements not only improves blood circulation, promoting the delivery of nutrients to the brain, but also stimulates the production of beneficial brain chemicals, fostering cognitive balance.

Women often find success in adopting exercise approaches that embrace gentleness and consistency. While the goal is to maintain physical activity as a lifelong companion, there is no need to engage in strenuous sessions. A regular routine of physical activity, even of short duration, can generate lasting results.

Activities such as dance, stretching, or tai chi can be versatile and enjoyable choices for women. These not only provide physical benefits but also offer a space for creative expression and relaxation, important elements in stress management and maintaining emotional balance.

Making exercise a lifelong companion thus becomes a wise choice for every woman eager to preserve and enhance her cognitive well-being. Through a ballet of measured movements, a woman can dance through life with an active, resilient, and vibrant brain.

Nurture Social and Intellectual Relationships

Research shows that those who engage in continuous learning and live in a socially rich environment have a lower risk of cognitive problems. Social interactions promote the production of neurotransmitters associated with well-being, helping to protect cognitive abilities.

Your mind is a social creature, shaped and strengthened by the web of relationships and intellectual challenges. Research clearly highlights that cultivating social and intellectual connections can be an elixir for your cognitive health.

Engaging in intellectual activities, such as studying, is a powerful ally in the fight against cognitive issues. Being part of an academic environment or committing to continuous learning reduces the risk of cognitive decline. This constant mental stimulation keeps your mind sharp and ready to tackle new challenges.

Social relationships are not just a pleasant aspect of life; they play a crucial role in protecting your cognitive abilities. Interacting with others stimulates the production of neurotransmitters like serotonin and oxytocin, which not only improve your mood but also help keep your brain active and resilient.

Participating in social groups, such as a book club or an intellectual circle, offers the dual reward of meaningful relationships and mental stimulation. Deep conversations and the sharing of ideas challenge your mind in a unique way, providing a workout for your intellect that protects your brain from the effects of aging.

In an increasingly digitally connected world, virtual sociality can be a valuable complement to physical interactions. Joining online communities, discussing topics of interest, and connecting with like-minded individuals can add an extra social and intellectual dimension to your life.

Nurturing social and intellectual relationships thus becomes a harmonious melody for your cognitive health. From academic studies to deep conversations, from social interactions to virtual connections, each note combines to create a symphony of mental well-being and brain resilience.

Manage Stress

Stress can radically alter hormones, inhibiting estrogen, which is essential for brain protection. Reducing stress in daily life has positive impacts on mental and cognitive health.

Stress acts as a powerful catalyst, triggering a cascade of hormonal changes in your body. Estrogen, essential for brain protection, can be inhibited by high levels of stress. Understanding this intricate interplay between stress and hormones is the first step in preserving brain health.

Chronic stress can cause significant damage to your mental and cognitive health. Prolonged exposure to high levels of cortisol, the stress hormone, can impair brain plasticity and interfere with memory and higher cognitive functions.

Managing stress, therefore, becomes a key strategy for balancing estrogen and preserving your brain. But how can you tackle stress in everyday life?

Embracing relaxation techniques, such as mindfulness meditation, deep breathing, or yoga, can be an effective way to reduce the effects of stress. These

 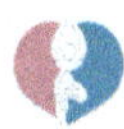

practices help lower cortisol levels and promote a relaxed response from the nervous system, thereby maintaining a healthy hormonal balance.

Introducing regenerative breaks into your day is essential. Even brief moments of relaxation, like a short walk or a break to enjoy some music, can help keep your brain in an optimal state.

Awareness of the sources of stress in your life is the first step to effectively addressing them. Honestly reflect on the situations or activities that generate stress and look for positive ways to manage them.

Managing stress thus becomes a self-protection strategy for your brain and overall well-being. Small changes in your daily routine, combined with an increasing awareness of stress sources, can make a difference in preserving estrogen and keeping your brain in optimal health.

Sleep Well to Live Well (see also Chapter 1)

Quality sleep is directly linked to hormonal balance. Less than 7-8 hours of sleep per day can cause hormonal imbalances, increasing the risk of neurological problems. Sleep is not just a period of rest; it is a fundamental element for maintaining hormonal balance and the optimal functioning of your brain. Let's explore the deep connection between quality sleep and your overall well-being.

During sleep, your body regulates the production of various hormones, influencing metabolism, growth, stress, and mood. Adequate levels of growth hormone and melatonin, for example, are crucial for cell regeneration and restorative sleep.

Chronic sleep deprivation, defined as less than 7-8 hours per day, can cause significant hormonal imbalances. Elevated levels of cortisol, the stress hormone, and a decrease in growth hormone release can result from insufficient sleep, increasing the risk of neurological problems and compromising your overall health.

Insomnia, often associated with hormonal disorders, can have a direct impact on the brain. Lack of sleep can contribute to cognitive problems, concentration difficulties, and mood disorders. Hormones involved in sleep regulation, when altered, can impair your ability to face daily challenges.

To improve sleep quality, maintain a consistent bedtime and wake-up schedule, even on non-working days. A regular routine helps synchronize your circadian rhythm, improving sleep quality.

 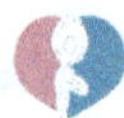

Ensure that your bedroom is a sanctuary for sleep. Darken the room, control the temperature, and reduce noise to create a favorable environment for rest.

Avoid caffeine and stimulants in the hours leading up to sleep. Reduce exposure to bright screens at least an hour before bed, as blue light can interfere with melatonin production.

Incorporate relaxation practices into your evening routine. Meditation, quiet reading, or a warm bath can mentally and physically prepare you for sleep.

Investing in your rest is not a luxury, but a necessity for your well-being. Maintaining quality sleep is an investment in your hormonal, mental, and physical health. Give yourself the necessary time for restorative sleep, and you will live each day with greater vitality and mental clarity.

Beware of Toxins (see also Chapter 10)

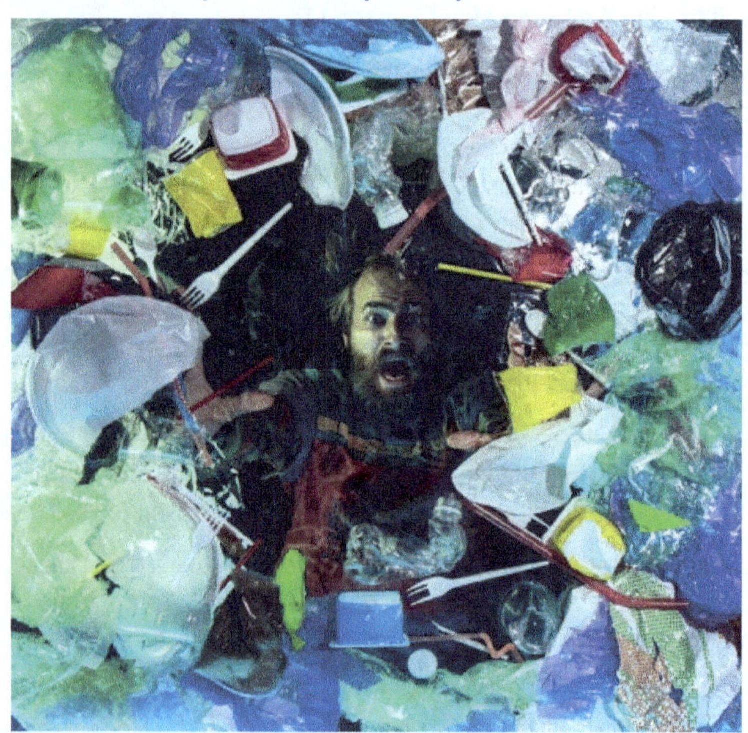

 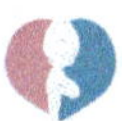

Reduce exposure to environmental toxins, such as BPA in plastic products. Choose organic foods, especially those eaten with the skin, to limit the intake of harmful substances.

Your daily dietary choices have a direct impact on your brain health. Genetics may play a minor role, but your lifestyle, diet, and habits profoundly influence your brain well-being.

Environmental toxins can significantly impact brain health. Reduce exposure to bisphenol A (BPA), commonly found in plastic products, by opting for safer alternatives. Use glass or stainless steel containers to reduce the risk of plastic contamination.

Choosing organic foods, especially those consumed with the skin, is a key strategy to limit the intake of harmful substances. Organic foods reduce exposure to pesticides and chemical fertilizers, providing your brain with nutrients without the harmful effects of chemical residues.

Your daily food choices are not just about satisfying hunger but profoundly impact your brain health. Genetics plays a marginal role compared to your lifestyle, diet, and habits.

Chemicals and toxins can enter the food chain and, subsequently, your body. The accumulation of these substances can contribute to neurological problems, compromising brain function and increasing the risk of long-term cognitive disorders.

In addition to avoiding harmful substances, focus on foods that promote brain health. Omega-3 fatty acids, found in fish, flaxseeds, and walnuts, are known to improve cognitive function. Antioxidants, present in berries and leafy green vegetables, can protect the brain from damage caused by free radicals.

Adopt a balanced diet rich in fruits, vegetables, whole grains, and lean proteins. Variety is key to ensuring you get all the essential nutrients to support optimal brain function.

Every time you choose what to put on your plate, you are making a direct choice for your brain health. Make these conscious choices a daily habit, as protecting your brain is a long-term investment in your quality of life.

 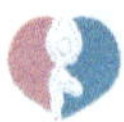

Chapter 13: "Hypertension Issues? Here's How to Solve Them"

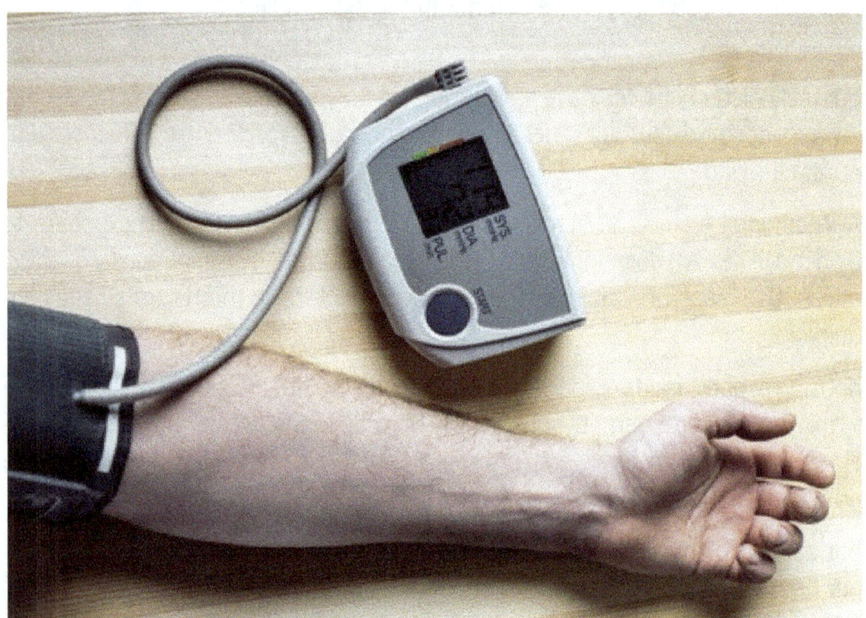

"We know how hypertension can be a serious problem, and often, its presence goes unnoticed due to the lack of obvious signs. It's almost like a 'silent killer' that could be lurking in our bodies. Doctors refer to it this way, and it can be frightening to think that what we don't see could affect our health so much.

When it comes to blood pressure, doctors recommend aiming for values around 120/80. This is a magic number that often eludes many of us. Surprisingly, one in three people in Italy finds themselves dealing with hypertension, with values higher than 130/80. It's more common than you might think, and you might even find yourself involved in this struggle without even knowing it.

Now, you might be wondering what you can do, right? How can you take care of your blood pressure without immediately resorting to complex solutions or medications that could have unwanted side effects?

Well, our chapter is right here to answer these questions. We don't want to scare you with data or complicated medical terms. We want to give you 15 natural remedies. These remedies are designed to lower blood pressure safely and gradually.

We'll explore together 12 strategies, starting from the simplest ones that can be easily integrated into your daily routine. I understand life can be complicated, and trying to manage health often seems like a daunting task. But don't worry, we're here to simplify things, step by step.

And you know what? We also want to debunk some common myths about blood pressure. For example, coffee isn't the enemy you might think, and quitting smoking is a wise step but not the only one. And excess salt? Well, it might not be exactly as you imagine.

So, take a moment, relax, and let this chapter guide you with practical advice. After all, your health is precious, and we're here to help you take care of it in the most natural way possible.

12 tips to help keep your blood pressure under control.

1.   Dark Chocolate:

Yes, you heard it right! Dark chocolate with at least 80% cocoa is a recommended treat. It contains flavonoids that fight inflammation, keeping your arteries healthy and flexible.

2. Garlic:

A small touch of raw garlic could make a difference. Studies suggest that garlic has anti-inflammatory and antifungal properties, helping to reduce blood pressure.

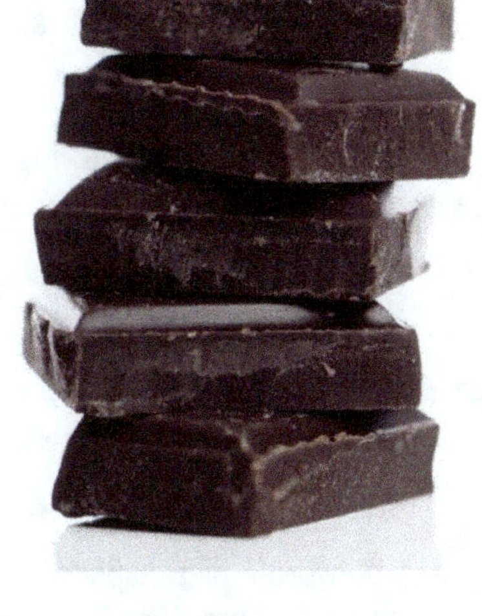

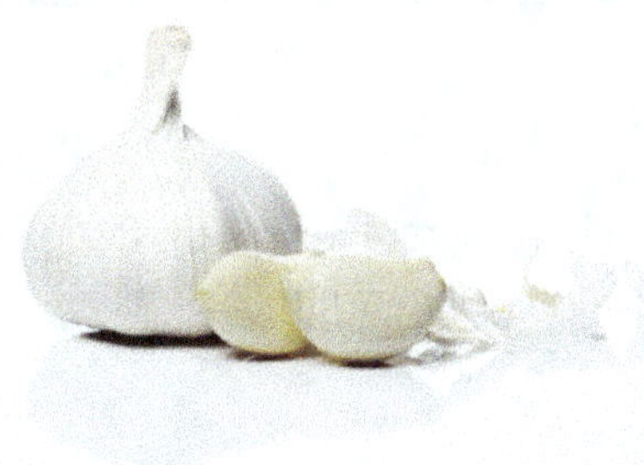

3. Protein in Your Diet:

Fish, meat, poultry, nuts, and legumes: they are all great allies in the fight against hypertension. However, keep an eye on kidney health, especially if you have kidney problems.

4. Omega-3s and Magnesium:

 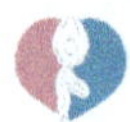

Fish, nuts, and other foods rich in omega-3s and magnesium can be valuable. You can also get them through a balanced diet or supplements.

5. Limiting Alcohol:

It's better to moderate alcohol consumption. Studies suggest that excess alcohol is linked to increased blood pressure.

6. Stress Management with Meditation:

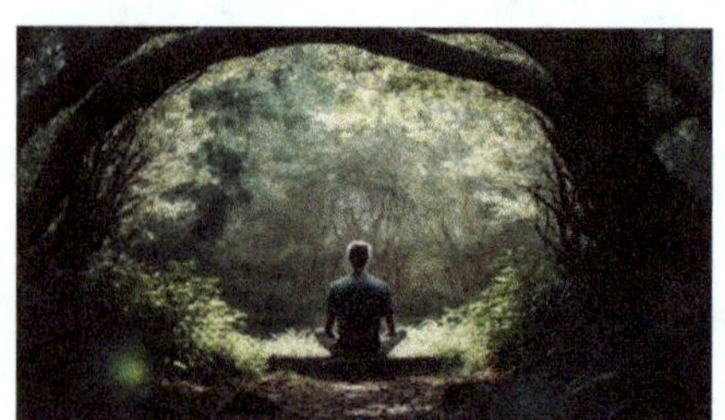

Meditation is like a breath of fresh air for your well-being. It helps reduce stress by lowering cortisol, the hormone that can affect your blood pressure.

7. Increase Potassium Intake:

A balanced diet rich in potassium can help lower blood pressure. Foods such as citrus fruits, salmon, chia seeds, and lentils are suggested to naturally supplement potassium.

8. Ensure Sufficient Sleep:

Lack of sleep can contribute to increased blood pressure. It's recommended to sleep between 8 and 9 hours each night to promote cardiovascular health.

9. Avoid Processed Foods:

Canned and processed foods, rich in preservatives and added sugars, can increase inflammation and blood pressure. It's advisable to prefer fresh, unprocessed foods.

10. Eliminate Refined Sugars and White Flour:

A low-carbohydrate diet, especially avoiding refined sugars and white flour, can help reduce blood pressure. It's emphasized that the main cause of arteriosclerosis is excess sugar.

11. Lose Weight:

Weight loss has an immediate impact on blood pressure. Intermittent fasting is also suggested as a means to promote satiety and weight control.

12. Regular Exercise:

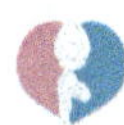

Regular physical activity is presented as the real remedy for many health problems, including hypertension. Even 10-15 minutes of physical activity per day can have significant benefits on blood pressure and overall health.

And now, I'd like to debunk three myths about blood pressure:

- Coffee: - Contrary to popular belief, coffee doesn't permanently increase blood pressure. Moderate consumption is generally considered safe.

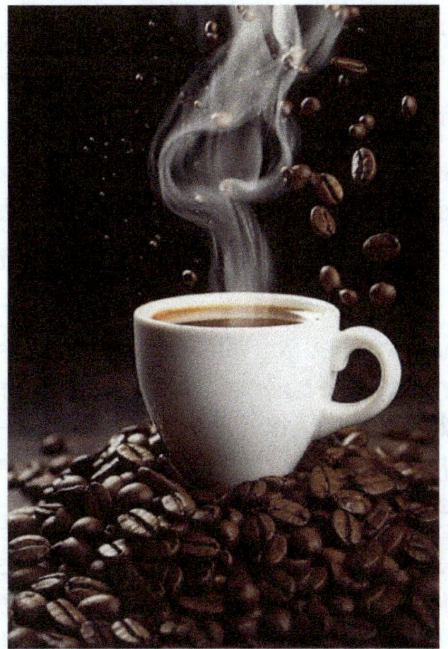

- Smoking: Although smoking may temporarily increase blood pressure, quitting is essential for overall health improvement.

- Excess Salt:

- Not everyone is affected by excess salt, but some people should limit their intake for specific health reasons.

These actions, combined with professional advice, can significantly contribute to maintaining balanced blood pressure and promoting your overall well-being. It's not just about treating symptoms but investing in your long-term health.

I hope these tips help you take care of your blood pressure naturally. Remember, small changes can make a big difference.

 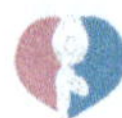

Conclusion

In this journey through your health and well-being, I hope you've found inspiration and valuable information to shape a more balanced and mindful life. Always remember that your health is a precious treasure, and every choice you make can influence your path to wellness. Whether you're starting a new chapter in your quest for a healthy life or deepening your knowledge, we're here to support you.

'Sana Vitae,' the way of health, is a commitment that lasts a lifetime. Every page of this book is an invitation to embrace conscious choices, adopt beneficial habits, and explore the healing power of nature. We hope you can apply this knowledge not only in your daily routine but also in your overall approach to existence.

Remember that your well-being is not just physical but also involves mind and spirit. Small daily actions can make a big difference in your journey of growth and self-realization. Start with small but consistent steps and allow change to deeply root in your life.

We hope this guide to natural wellness has provided you with valuable insights and inspiration to embark on a healthier and more balanced life journey. Your opinion is crucial to us, as is your health. We invite you to share your experience and reflections on this book through an honest review. Your words can inspire others to embark on their journey to 'Sana Vitae.'

Thank you for being part of our wellness and mindfulness community. Your voice matters, and we are grateful for every thought you wish to share. Together, we can build a path of growth and health for all.

Thank you for choosing to purchase the first volume of the 'Sana Vitae' series. May you live a balanced, mindful, and fulfilling life. May you find joy in daily choices, in balancing mind, body, and spirit. Your health is a continuous journey, and we are honored to be part of your path to lasting wellness. Start today, because your health is the greatest gift you can give yourself.

www.ingramcontent.com/pod-product-compliance
Lightning Source LLC
Chambersburg PA
CBHW071503030726
47593CB00003B/1135